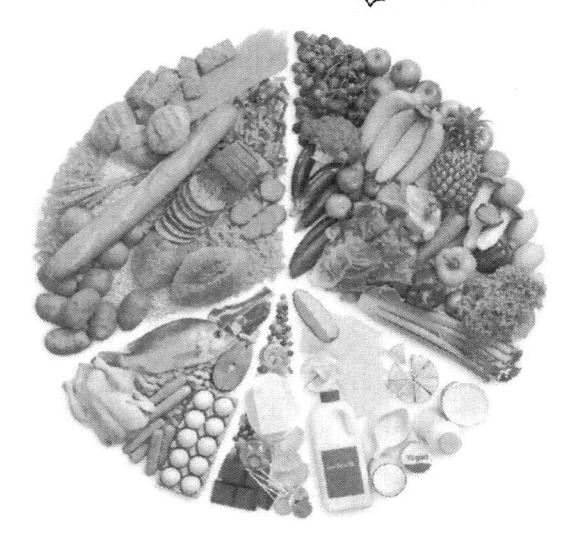

DASH DIET FOR BEGINNERS

The practical guide to improving blood pressure and losing weight with recipes and the 21-Day Dash Diet meal plan.

MERILYN HELLIS

DISCLAIMER

This book contains neither medical advice nor prescriptions of any treatment technique for diseases, disorders, pathologies and does not replace medical advice. The author's goal is to provide explanations and useful information for your personal search for well-being, both physical and emotional. The author declines all responsibility.

All rights reserved. The text and parts of it cannot be disclosed, stored, transmitted to third parties or copied without having received authorization from the author.

The registered trademarks used have no consent and the publication of the registered trademark is without authorization or approval of the registered trademark owner. All trademarks and registered trademarks within this book are for clarification purposes only and are the property of the owners themselves, not affiliated with this document.

TABLE OF CONTENTS

THE ORIGINS OF THE DASH DIET 1
What Does This Diet Include?..8

Clinical Significance...12

Enhancing Healthcare Team Outcomes 13

SIMPLE RECIPES TO REDISCOVER YOUR SHAPE.. 15

Breakfast Dishes 15

   Homemade Greek-Style Yogurt......................................15

   Serves:..15

   Ingredients:..16

   Banana-Nut Oatmeal..18

   Serves:..18

   Ingredients:..18

   Apple-Cinnamon Baked Oatmeal 20

   Servings:...20

   Ingredients:..20

   Breakfast Casserole 22

   Servings:...22

   Ingredients:..22

Lunch Dishes 24

   Chili 24

   Serves:..24

   Ingredients:..24

Cooking Instructions: 24

Corn Tamales with Avocado-Tomatillo Salsa 26

Serves: 26

Ingredients: 26

Cooking Instructions: 27

Buffalo Chicken Salad Wrap 28

Ingredients: 28

Cooking Instructions: 28

Pasta Salad with Mixed Vegetables 29

Serves: 29

Ingredients: 29

Cooking Instructions: 29

Soft Tacos with Southwestern Vegetables 31

Serves: 31

Ingredients: 31

Cooking Instructions: 31

Tuna Pita Pockets 33

Serves: 33

Ingredients: 33

Cooking Instructions: 33

Serves: 34

Ingredients: 34

Cooking Instructions: 35

Dinner Soups 36

Chicken Broth	36
Servings:	36
Ingredients:	36
Potato Leek Soup with Beans	38
Serves:	38
Ingredients:	38
Cooking Instructions:	39
Crockpot French Onion Soup	41
Serves:	41
Ingredients:	41
Slow Cooker Chicken Noodle Soup	43
Serves:	43
Ingredients:	43
Hearty Minestrone Soup	45
Serves:	45
Ingredients:	45
New England Clam Chowder	47
Serves:	47
Ingredients:	47
Crock-Pot Lobster Bisque	49
Serves:	49
Ingredients:	49
Meatball Soup	52
Serves:	52

Ingredients: 52

Chicken Tortilla Soup 54

Serves: 54

Ingredients: 54

Corn and Shrimp Chowder 56

Serves: 56

Ingredients: 56

Split Pea Soup 58

Serves: 58

Ingredients: 58

Poultry Dishes 60

Mexican Chicken Stew 60

Serves: 60

Ingredients: 60

Crockpot Chicken Fajitas 62

Serves: 62

Ingredients: 62

Black Bean Chicken 64

Serves: 64

Ingredients: 64

Cooking Instructions: 64

Turkey Chili 66

Serves: 66

Ingredients: 66

Mediterranean Roast Turkey Breast 68
Serves: 68
Ingredients: 68
Honey-Glazed Chicken Wings 70
Serves: 70
Ingredients: 70
Jambalaya 72
Serves: 72
Ingredients: 72
Slow-Cooker Turkey Stroganoff 74
Serves: 74
Ingredients: 74
Provencal Chicken and White Beans 76
Serves: 76
Ingredients: 76
White Chicken Chili 78
Serves: 78
Ingredients: 78

Desserts 80
Slow Cooker Brown Rice Pudding 80
Serves: 80
Ingredients: 80
Berry Cobbler 82
Serves: 82

Ingredients: 82

Spiced Apple Sauce 84

Serves: 84

Ingredients: 84

Apple Crisp 86

Serves: 86

Meat Dishes (Beef, Pork, Lamb, Veal) 88

Barbecued Pork 88

Serves: 88

Ingredients: 88

Slow Cooker Chili 90

Serves: 90

Ingredients: 90

Cooking Instructions: 90

Spaghetti Sauce with Meat and Vegetables 92

Serves: 92

Ingredients: 92

Slow Cooker Bolognese Sauce 94

Serves: 94

Ingredients: 94

Mexican Beef Stew 96

Serves: 96

Ingredients: 96

Moroccan Beef Tagine 98

- Serves: 98
- Ingredients: 98
- Lamb Tagine with Pears 100
- Serves: 100
- Ingredients: 100
- Slow-Cooker Beef Stew Provencal 102
- Serves: 102
- Ingredients: 102
- Slow-Cooked Beef Roast 104
- Serves: 104
- Ingredients: 104
- Beef Stew with Butternut Squash 106
- Serves: 106
- Ingredients: 106
- Irish Stew 108
- Serves: 108
- Ingredients: 108
- Serves: 109
- Ingredients: 109

Vegetable Dishes 111
- Baked Potatoes with Broccoli and Mushrooms 111
- Serves: 111
- Ingredients: 111
- Sweet Potato Coconut Curry 113

Serves: 113

Ingredients: 113

Mediterranean Vegetable Stew 114

Serves: 114

Ingredients: 114

Slow Cooker Baked Beans 115

Serves: 115

Moroccan Root Vegetable Tagine 116

Serves: 116

Ingredients: 116

Vegetarian Vegetable Stew 117

Serves: 117

Ingredients: 117

WHAT TO EAT, WHEN AND IN WHAT QUANTITIES? 118

Vegetables: 119

Fruits: 119

Low-fat dairy foods: 119

Meat, fish, poultry: 119

Nuts, seeds, and beans: 119

Fats and oils: 119

Sweets: 120

Precautions 121

Risks 122

What is the recommended daily allowance of sodium? 123

How does the DASH diet lower blood pressure and promote weight loss? 123

DASH Diet and Weight Loss: How to Cut Calories From Your Day 124

Breakfast: 128

Morning snack: 128

Lunch: 128

Afternoon snack: 128

Dinner: 128

Dessert: 128

What are some DASH diet recipes? 129

Breakfast 129

Lunch 129

Dinner 130

Snacks 130

How can I make the DASH diet tastier? 130

What heart-healthy lifestyle interventions are part of the DASH diet? 131

Physical activity, weight loss and high blood pressure. 131

Weight management and high blood pressure 132

Alcohol use and high blood pressure 133

Stress management and high blood pressure 133

Sleep and high blood pressure 134

Smoking and high blood pressure 134

HOW TO LOSE WEIGHT IN SEVEN DAYS BY EATING 136

Phase 1: Two Weeks to Lose Weight by Eating 136

Phase 2: Kick It Up a Notch! 137

Whole Grains: 138

Fruit: 138

Low-Fat Milk or Yogurt: 138

Sugar: 138

Alcohol: 138

Phase 1: 7 Days to Lose Weight by Eating 138

Day 1 138

Breakfast 138

Lunch 139

Mid-Afternoon Snack 139

Before-Dinner Snack (Optional) 139

Dinner 140

Day 2 141

Breakfast 141

Mid-Morning Snack 141

Lunch 141

Mid-Afternoon Snack 142

Dinner 142

Day 3 143

Breakfast 143

Mid-Morning Snack 143

Lunch 143

Mid-Afternoon Snack 144

Dinner 144

Day 5 145

Breakfast 145

Mid-Morning Snack (Optional) 145

Lunch 145

Mid-Afternoon Snack 145

Before-Dinner Snack (Optional) 145

Dinner 146

Day 6 147

Breakfast 147

Mid-Morning Snack (Optional) 147

Lunch 147

Mid-Afternoon Snack 148

Dinner 148

Day 7 149

Breakfast 149

Mid-Morning Snack (Optional) 149

Lunch 149

Mid-Afternoon Snack 149

Before-Dinner Snack (Optional) 150

Dinner 150

EMPTY THE PANTRY AND CHANGE EATING HABITS 152

Motivation to Change: 152

Cleaning Out the Kitchen: 153

Grocery Guide: 155

1. The First Thing You Need to Do Before You Go Shopping is Prepare. 155

2. Remember What the DASH Diet is All About. 156

3. Keep DASH Diet-Friendly Items in the House. 157

4. Choose Your Cookware. 159

5. Be Aware of Healthy Cooking Practices. 159

DASH Diet Food List 160

Fruits and Vegetables: 160

Whole Grains: 161

Dairy: 161

Legumes, Nuts, and Seeds: 161

Oils: 161

HOW TO PREPARE/ DEFEAT MENOPAUSAL KILOGRAMS WITH THE DASH DIET 162

EAT THIS 163

AVOID THESE 165

HOW TO LOSE 10 CENTIMETERS OF WAISTLINE IN 21 DAYS 168

What Causes Waistline Fat for Women in Menopause? 168
Stress 169
Dealing with Stress 170
Insulin 172
21-Day Activities to Lose 10 Centimeters of Fat Waistline 173
Day 1 173
DASH Recipe: 173
Workout: 173
Day 2 174
DASH Recipe: 174
Workout: 174
Day 3 174
DASH Recipe: 174
Workouts: 175
Day 4 175
DASH Recipe: 175
Workouts: 176
Day 5 176
DASH Recipe: 176
Workout: 176
Day 6 177
DASH Recipes: 177
Workouts: 177

- Day 7 177
- DASH Recipe: 177
- Workout: 178
- Day 8 178
- DASH Recipe: 178
- Workout: 178
- Day 9 179
- DASH Recipe: 179
- Day 10 180
- Workout: 180
- Day 11 181
- DASH Recipe: 181
- Workout: 181
- Day 12 181
- DASH Recipe: 181
- Workout: 181
- Day 13 182
- DASH Recipe: 182
- Workout: 182
- Day 14 183
- Workout: 183
- Day 15 184
- DASH Recipe: 184
- Workout: 184

Day 16	184
DASH Recipe:	184
Workout:	185
Day 17	185
DASH Recipe:	185
Workout:	185
Day 18	186
DASH Recipe:	186
Workouts:	186
Day 19	187
DASH Recipe:	187
Workout:	187
Day 20	188
Workout:	188
Day 21	188
DASH Recipe:	188
Workout:	189
Fighting Waistline Fat With the DASH Diet	189
The Five Principles to a Successful Nutrition Plan	190
What to Eat	191
Fruits and Vegetables	192
Beans and Legumes	196
Meat and Fish	196
Additional Ingredients	197

What Not to Eat 201

Drink Recipes to Lose Waistline Fat for Women in Menopause 204

Fighting Waistline Fat with the DASH Diet + Exercises 206

The Home Workout.. 207

The Crunch 207

The Plank 208

Scissors 209

The Routine 210

Take up Pilates 211

CONCLUSION 213

REFERENCES 216

THE ORIGINS OF THE DASH DIET

It has been discovered that high blood pressure distresses about one in three adults in the United States, and is defined as blood pressure consistently above 140/90mmHg. The high number, 140, is the systolic pressure exerted by the blood against the arteries while the heart is contracting. The low number, 90, is the diastolic pressure in the arteries while the heart is relaxing or between beats. The concern is the higher the blood pressure, the greater the risk for developing heart disease, kidney disease, and stroke. High blood pressure is known as the silent killer as it has no symptoms or warning signs.

Over the last 50 years in the United States, clinicians have seen a rise in diseases including hypertension (HTN), diabetes, obesity, and coronary artery disease (CAD). It is estimated that around 2000 people die of heart disease every day in the United States. Chronic diseases related to diet and obesity have become major causes of death in the United States across all ethnicities. Obesity has been linked to the major etiological factor in diabetes, HTN, cancer, and CAD.

Although there have been several advancements in the scientific world regarding new medications and cutting-edge diagnostic techniques, the rate of these diseases has multiplied many times. This increase has been at a particularly high rate in the last 20 years. Due to this trend, major organizations including the American Heart Association, National Institutes of Health, and National Heart, Lung, and Blood Institute, have all started looking at an integrative approach to managing this growing epidemic. Diagnostic testing and medications are still the mainstays of patient management. However, the importance of diet, exercise, stress reduction, and lifestyle habits cannot be ignored.

Studies over the years have advocated that high intakes of salt play a role in the development of high blood pressure. Dietary advice for the prevention and lowering of high blood pressure has focused primarily on reducing sodium or salt intake. A 1989 study looked at the response an intake of 3–12g of salt per day had on blood pressure. The study found that modest reductions in salt, of 5–6 g salt per day, caused blood pressures to fall in people with hypertension. The best effect was seen with only 3g of salt per day, with blood pressure decreasing by an average of 11 mmHg systolic and 6mmHg diastolic. More recently, the use of low-salt diets for the prevention or treatment of high blood pressure has come into question. The Trials of Hypertension Prevention Phase II in 1997 indicated that energy intake and weight loss were more important than the restriction of dietary salt in the prevention of hypertension. A 2006 review from Cochrane, which looked at the effect of longer-term modest salt reduction on blood pressure, found that modest reductions in salt intake could have a significant effect on blood pressure for those with high blood pressure, but a lesser effect on those without it. It was agreed that the 2007 public health recommendations of reducing salt intake from levels of 9–12g/day to a moderate 5–6g/day would have a favorable effect on blood pressure and cardiovascular disease. The effectiveness of the DASH diet for lowering blood pressure has been well recognized. The 2015 Dietary Guidelines for Americans recommend the DASH Eating Plan as an example of a balanced eating plan, consistent with the existing guidelines, and it forms the basis for the USDA MyPlate. DASH is also recommended in other guidelines, such as those advocated by the British Nutrition Foundation, American Heart Association, and American Society for Hypertension.

Although reducing sodium and increasing potassium, calcium, and magnesium intake play a key role in lowering blood pressure, the reasons the DASH eating plan have a beneficial effect remain uncertain. The researchers suggest it may be because whole foods improve the absorption of the potassium, calcium, and magnesium, or it may be related to the cumulative effect of eating these nutrients together rather than the individual nutrients themselves. It is also speculated that it may be something else in the fruits, vegetables, and low-fat dairy products that accounts for the association between the diet and blood pressure.

The Salt Institute supports the DASH diet but without the salt restriction. They claim that the DASH diet alone, without reduced sodium intake from manufactured foods, would achieve the desired blood pressure reduction. Their recommendation is based on the fact that there are no evidence-based studies supporting the need for dietary salt restriction for the entire population. The Cochrane review in 2006 showed that modest reductions in salt intake lower blood pressure significantly in people with hypertension, but have less of an effect on individuals with normal blood pressure. Restriction of salt for those without hypertension is not recommended. The DASH study by the National Heart, Lung, and Blood Institute (NHLBI), published in the New England Journal of Medicine in 1977, was the first study to look at the effect a diet rich in potassium, magnesium, and calcium, without supplements, had on blood pressure.

The study involved 459 adults with and without high blood pressure. Systolic blood pressures needed to be lower than 160 mmHg, and diastolic pressures between 80 and 95 mmHg. Approximately half the participants were women and 60% were African American. Three eating plans were compared. The first was similar to a typical American diet—high in fat (37% of calories) and low in fruit and vegetables. The second was a typical American diet but with more fruits and vegetables. The third was a plan rich in fruits, vegetables, low-fat dairy foods, and low in overall fat (less than 30% of calories). It also provided 4,700 milligrams (mg) potassium, 500mg magnesium, and 1,240 mg calcium per 2,000 calories. This has become known as the DASH diet. All three plans contained equal amounts of sodium, about 3,000mg of sodium daily, equivalent to 7 grams (g) of salt. This was approximately 20% below the average intake for adults in the United States, and close to the current salt recommendations of 4–5g daily. Calorie intake was adjusted to maintain each person's weight. These two factors were included to eliminate salt reduction and weight loss as potential reasons for any changes in blood pressure. All meals were prepared for the participants in a central kitchen, to increase compliance with the diets.

Results showed that the increased fruit and vegetable and DASH plans lowered blood pressure, but the DASH plan was the most effective in doing this. For participants without high blood pressure, it reduced systolic pressure by 6 mmHg and diastolic pressure by 3 mmHg. The results were better for participants with high blood pressure—the drop in systolic and diastolic was almost double, at 11mmHg and 6mmHg, respectively. These results showed that the DASH diet appeared to lower blood pressure as well as a

3g salt-restricted diet, but more importantly, had a similar reduction to that seen with the use of a single blood pressure medication. The effect was seen within two weeks of starting the DASH plan, which is also comparable to treatment by medication, and it was continued throughout the trial. This trial provided the first experimental evidence that potassium, calcium, and magnesium were important dietary factors in affecting blood pressure, rather than just sodium alone.

A typical modern American diet is high in saturated fats, omega 6 fatty acids, high glycemic load carbohydrates, and many artificial additives. This unhealthy diet combined with little training in nutrition among the medical professionals is being considered a major setback in tackling these diseases. Fortunately, there has been tremendous amount of research done in the last few decades into examining the effects of dietary patterns on chronic diseases, and this information is widely available to physicians online. Use of the Dietary Approaches to Stop Hypertension (DASH) diet began in the 1990s, and in 1992, the National Institutes of Health (NIH) started carrying out research projects to see if specific dietary interventions were useful in treating hypertension. Subjects included in the study were advised to follow just the dietary interventions and not include any other lifestyle modifications, in order to avoid any confounding factors. They found that just the dietary intervention alone was able to decrease systolic blood pressure by about 6 to 11mmHg. This effect was seen both in hypertensive (high blood pressure) as well as normotensive (normal blood pressure) people. Based on these results, in some instances DASH has been advocated as the first line pharmacologic therapy along with lifestyle modification.

What Does This Diet Include? Simply, DASH promotes the consumption of vegetables and fruits, lean meat and dairy products and the inclusion of micronutrients in the diet. It also advocates the reduction of sodium in the diet to about 1500mg/day. The DASH diet emphasizes the consumption of minimally processed and fresh food, and it has many similarities to some of the other dietary patterns which are promoted for cardiovascular health. In some respects, the DASH diet is a culmination of the ancient and modern world. It has been devised by scientists based on certain ancient dietary principles and has been tailored to target some of the leading killers of the modern society.

A typical serving guide for a patient following the DASH diet is as follows:

- Vegetables: about 5 servings per day.
- Fruits: about 5 servings per day.
- Carbohydrates: about 7 servings per day.
- Low-fat dairy products: about 2 servings per day.
- Lean meat products: about 2 or fewer servings per day.
- Nuts and seeds: 2 to 3 times per week.

Following is a closer look at these recommendations.

Carbohydrates in the diet are mainly composed of cellulose and starches, though the human body cannot digest cellulose which is mainly present in plant fiber. Healthy starches or carbohydrates have to be included in the diet, not only for the energy they can represent but also for the protective micronutrients. Low-carbohydrate diets are not necessarily healthy as they may lead to either an decreased caloric intake than is recommended, or a consumption of unhealthy fats as a substitute.

Healthy carbohydrates included under DASH include:

- Green leafy vegetables: kale, broccoli, spinach, collards, mustards.
- Whole grains: cracked wheat, millets, oats.
- Low-glycemic index fruits.
- Legumes and beans.
- Fats.

Fats have been considered a negative influence until now, in the development of the chronic disease epidemic. However, research has now shown otherwise, and fats are now classified as good fats and bad fats.

Good fats prevent inflammation, provide essential fatty acids and promote overall health. These fats, when consumed in moderation, have shown an increase in HDL and a lowering of small dense LDL particles. Some of the sources of good fats also included in the DASH diet include:

- Olive oil
- Avocados
- Nuts

- Hempseeds
- Flax seeds
- Fish rich in omega 3 fatty acids

Bad fats which include margarine, vegetable shortenings, partially hydrogenated vegetable oils, can cause an increase in small LDL particles, which promote atherogenesis.

Fats are a highly condensed source of energy and therefore have to be consumed in moderation. The serving sizes are much smaller than those of other nutrients on the DASH diet recommendations.

The DASH diet recommends more servings of plant proteins like legumes, soy products, nuts, and seeds.

Animal protein in the diet should mainly be composed of lean meats, low-fat dairy, eggs, and fish.

Processed and cured meats are not recommended as they have been shown to cause hypertension and also contain carcinogens.

The DASH diet also talks about the inclusion of certain foods which are rich in potassium, calcium, and magnesium, as these prevent endothelial dysfunction and promote endothelial, smooth muscle relaxation. Some of the foods rich in potassium include bananas, oranges, and spinach. Calcium is rich in dairy products and green leafy vegetables. Magnesium is present in a variety of whole grains, leafy vegetables, nuts, and seeds.

Clinical Significance

Is the DASH diet exclusively preferred only for treating HTN?

Since the formulation of the DASH diet program, it has been studied extensively to look for the effects on various other diseases.

Several studies have shown that the DASH diet helps lower blood glucose levels, triglycerides, LDL-C, and insulin resistance. This makes the DASH diet a very important adjunct to pharmacological therapy in metabolic syndromes, a major epidemic in this country. It also has been a successful tool in weight management. In certain populations, adherence to the DASH diet has shown significant improvements in the control of type 2 diabetes. It is a preferred diet in patients with heart failure, due to its emphasis on the reduction of dietary sodium and encouraging the intake of potassium, magnesium, and calcium.

The DASH diet has also shown a reduction in the incidence of colorectal cancer, mainly in white populations. The diet has also been proven in multiple studies to have lowered all-cause mortality in adults.

Based on these studies, it is safe to say that when combined with pharmacological intervention, the DASH diet can be a very useful tool for physicians to tackle these diseases more efficiently. When compared to some other diet patterns, it has an added advantage of having clear guidelines on the serving sizes and food groups, which makes it easier for physicians to prescribe and monitor their patients' improvement.

Enhancing Healthcare Team Outcomes

The DASH diet is a nutritionally-based approach to prevent and control hypertension. The diet has been tested in several clinical trials and has been shown to lower cholesterol, saturated fats, and blood pressure. The DASH diet has been recommended as the best diet to help people who would like to lose and maintain a healthy weight, and also lower blood pressure. The key issue is that this diet needs to be promoted to patients, and aside from physicians, both nurses and pharmacists play a key role in educating patients about the benefits of the diet. This is because prior to discharge, nurses are in a prime position to educate all patients and their families about the DASH diet and its benefits. Similarly, when patients visit a pharmacy, the pharmacist should educate the patient about the DASH diet. The most important feature about the DASH diet is it requires a change in lifestyle and adopt a healthy way to eat. In addition, patients should be encouraged to stop smoking, abstain from alcohol and do some type of physical activity on a regular basis.

The DASH diet has been well studied in many clinical trials, and in most of them has been associated with the lowering of blood pressure. Further, there is evidence to show that the DASH diet also lowers the risk of adverse cardiac events, stroke, type 2 diabetes, and obesity. Unfortunately, compliance to the diet remains low, and beyond clinical trials there are limited studies into the long-term effectiveness of the DASH diet.

SIMPLE RECIPES TO REDISCOVER YOUR SHAPE

Breakfast Dishes

Homemade Greek-Style Yogurt

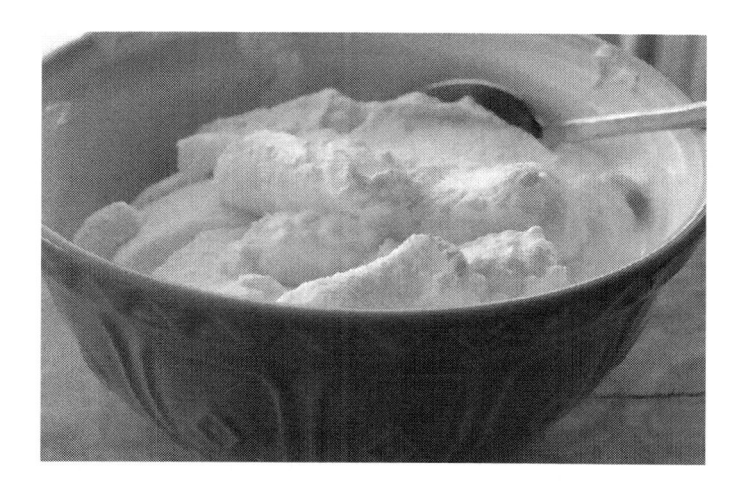

If you eat a lot of yogurt then you know it can be expensive. Making your own is really simple with the help of a slow cooker.

Serves: 8 (1 cup size)

Ingredients: ½ gallon 2 percent milk, 1 cup powdered milk (this is optional but does make the yogurt thicker), ½ cup live yogurt culture (can use regular plain yogurt). A thermometer, a small blanket, and a cheesecloth for straining are also needed.

Cooking Instructions:

1. Pour milk into a slow cooker. Stir in powdered milk. Heat the milk in the slow cooker on high until it reaches 180°F (about 1-2 hours depending on your cooker). Turn off the slow cooker and let the milk cool to around 110°F. Stir in the live yogurt culture and mix until completely blended. Wrap the slow cooker (which is turned off) in a blanket to keep the heat in. Let it sit for 6-8 hours.
2. Take lid off the slow cooker. To make thick, Greek-style yogurt you will need to drain the whey (the liquid on top of the yogurt) out of the yogurt. To do this, place a few layers of cheesecloth in a colander. Place the colander over a large bowl. Add the yogurt to the colander and let it drain in the refrigerator for a couple

of hours until it has reached the desired consistency.
3. Pour the yogurt into mason jars (or other containers) and store in the refrigerator for 7-10 days.

Nutritional Information (per serving): Calories 143, total fat 3.5g, sodium 159mg, total carbohydrates 19 g, dietary fiber 0 g, protein 18 g.

Banana-Nut Oatmeal

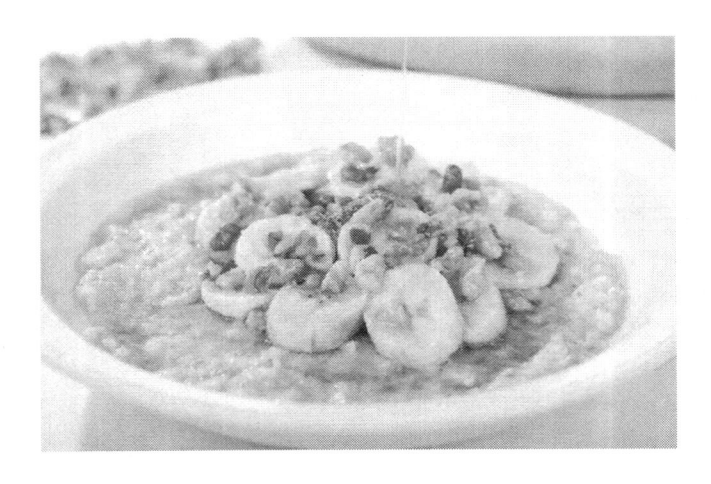

Another tasty version of oatmeal that will be ready for you when you wake up in the morning.

Serves: 4

Ingredients: 1 cup steel cut oats, 1 banana, mashed, ⅓ cup walnuts (chopped), 2 cups skim milk, 2 cups water, ⅓ cup honey, 2 teaspoons cinnamon, ½ teaspoon nutmeg, 1 teaspoon vanilla extract, ½ teaspoon salt

Cooking Instructions:

1. Place all ingredients in slow cooker. Stir well, cover, and cook at a low heat for 8 hours.

2. Serve with extra banana slices and walnuts on top.

Nutritional Information (per serving): Calories 310, sodium 365 mg, protein 11g, carbohybrates 42g, dietary fiber 6g, fat 9g.

Apple-Cinnamon Baked Oatmeal

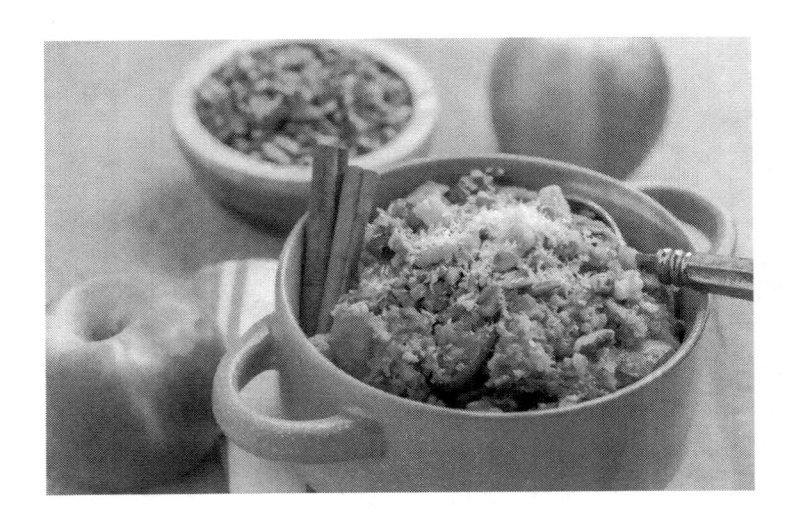

This oatmeal recipe is cooked in the slow cooker so you can wake up to a warm and satisfying breakfast without any fuss.

Servings: 8

Ingredients: 2 cups steel cut oats, 8 cups water, 1 teaspoon cinnamon, ½ teaspoon allspice, ½ teaspoon nutmeg, ¼ cup brown sugar, 1 teaspoon vanilla extract, 2 apples, diced, 1 cup raisins, ½ cup unsalted, roasted walnuts (chopped).

Cooking Instructions:

1. Spray slow cooker with nonstick cooking spray.
2. Add all the ingredients to the slow cooker except for the walnuts. Mix well to combine.
3. Set slow cooker to low setting and cook for 8 hours.
4. Serve topped with chopped walnuts

Nutritional Information (per serving): Calories 312, sodium 4mg, protein 9g, carbohydrates 60g, fat 7.5 g, sugar 23g.

Note: Be sure to use steel cut oats for this recipe, and not instant or rolled oats, or you may end up with a sticky mess.

Breakfast Casserole

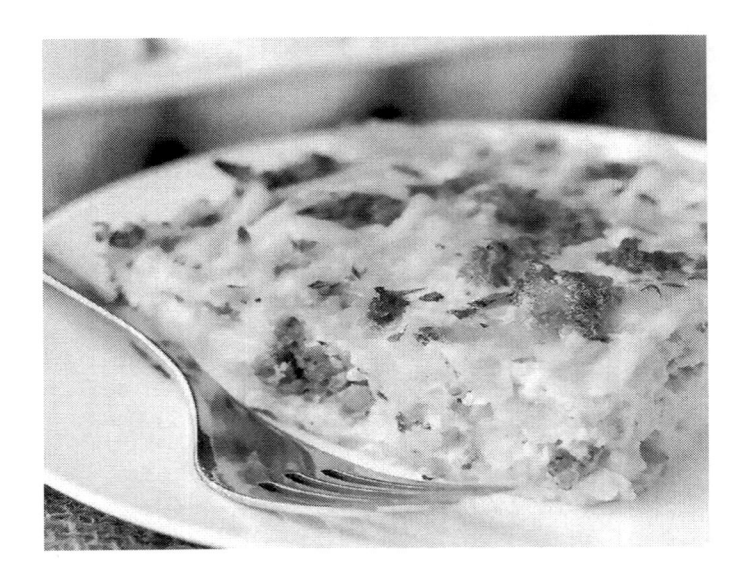

Perfect for a relaxing Sunday brunch.

Servings: 8

Ingredients: 4 cups frozen hash browns, 12 eggs, ½ cup low-fat milk, 10 ounces low-sodium sausage (cooked), 8 ounces cheddar cheese (shredded), 2 garlic cloves (minced), 1 medium onion (diced), ½ red bell pepper (diced), freshly ground black pepper.

Cooking Instructions:

1. Spray bottom of a slow cooker with cooking spray.

2. Crack eggs into large bowl. Add milk, mustard, and black pepper, and whisk until combined.
3. Spread ½ hash browns on bottom of the slow cooker. Top each with half the sausage, cheese, garlic, onion, and bell pepper. Add a second layer with hash browns, sausage, cheese, garlic, onion, and bell pepper.
4. Pour the egg mixture over layers. Cover, and cook on low setting for 4 to 5 hours, or on high for 2 to 3 hours, until the eggs are set.

Nutritional Information (per serving): Calories 336, total fat 23g, sodium 468mg, total carbs 13g, protein 19g.

Lunch Dishes

Chili

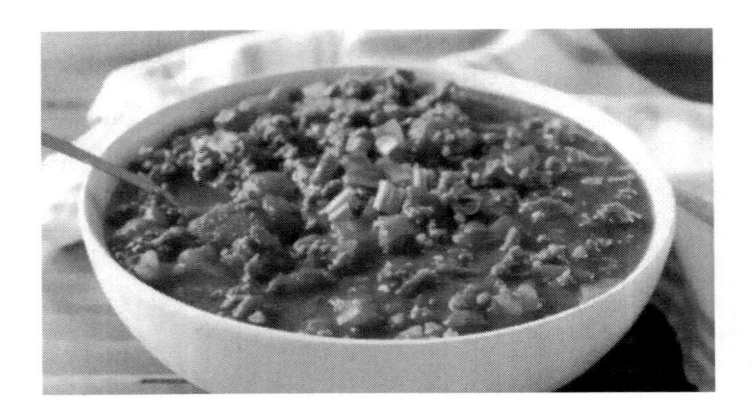

Serves: 8

Ingredients: 1 pound extra-lean ground beef, ½ cup chopped onion, 2 large tomatoes (or 2 cups canned, unsalted tomatoes), 4 cups canned kidney beans, rinsed and drained, 1 cup chopped celery, 1 teaspoon sugar, 1½ tablespoons chili powder or water to taste, 2 tablespoons cornmeal Jalapeno peppers, (seeded and chopped).

Cooking Instructions: In a large pot add onions and ground beef. Sauté meat until browned and onion is cooked. Drain. Add beans, tomatoes, celery, chili powder, and sugar to beef mixture. Cook covered for 10 minutes. Make sure to stir. Add water and stir in cornmeal. Cook for an additional 10 minutes.

Corn Tamales with Avocado-Tomatillo Salsa

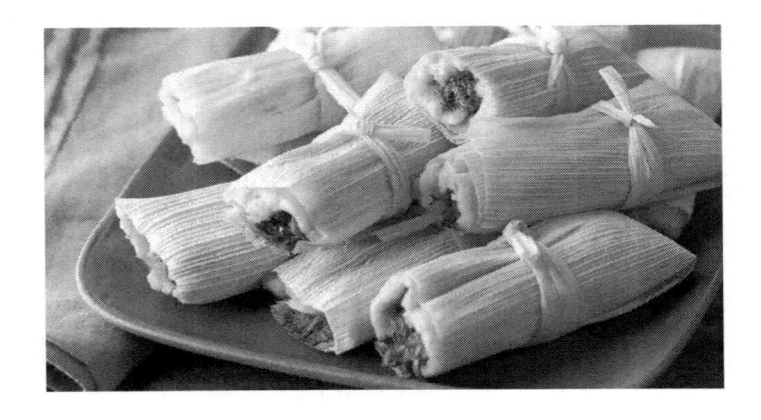

Serves: 6

Ingredients: 18 dried corn husks (plus extra husks to make ties), 3 cups fresh corn kernels or frozen kernels (thawed), 2 cups masa harina, ½ cup lukewarm water, 1 teaspoon baking powder, ½ teaspoon salt, 3 tablespoons canola oil, ¼ cup diced red bell pepper (capsicum), ¼ cup diced green bell pepper (capsicum), 2 tablespoons diced yellow onion, ⅛ teaspoon red pepper flakes. For the salsa ¼ cup chopped avocado, 5 ounces tomatillos (husked under warm running water and chopped), 1 tablespoon fresh lime juice, 2 tablespoons chopped fresh cilantro or fresh coriander, ½ teaspoon seeded, minced jalapeno chili, ¼ teaspoon salt.

Cooking Instructions: Soften corn husks in a bowl of water for 10 minutes. Rinse, drain and pat dry.

Puree 2½ cups of corn in food processor. Combine masa harina, pureed corn, water, salt, oil and baking powder in a large bowl.

Cook in a nonstick frying pan. Add the onion, bell peppers, and remaining corn. Sauté until cooked for about 7-8 minutes. To make the tamale, put 3 tablespoons of masa mixture in the corn husk. Flatten and make a well in the center. Add 1 tablespoon vegetables. Fold and tie with strip of torn husk. Boil two inches of water in a pot with a steamer basket. Layer the tamales in the basket. Cover with a towel and steam for an hour. Make salsa by combining tomatillos, lime, cilantro, avocado, and jalapeño with ¼ teaspoon of salt.

Buffalo Chicken Salad Wrap

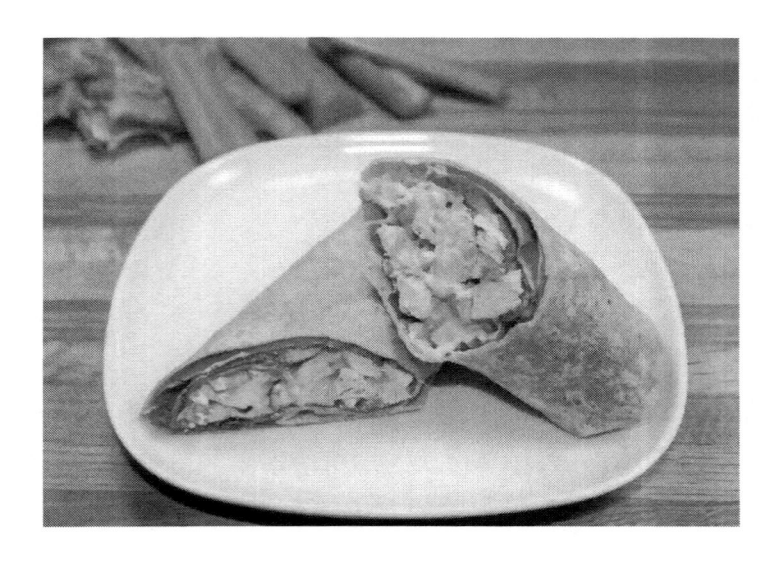

Ingredients: 3-4 ounces of chicken breasts, 2 whole chipotle peppers, ¼ cup white wine vinegar, ¼ cup low-calorie mayonnaise, 2 stalks celery, 2 carrots (diced, cut into matchsticks), 1 small yellow onion (diced about ½ cup), ½ cup thinly sliced rutabaga or other root vegetable, 4 ounces spinach (cut into strips), 2 whole-grain tortillas (12-inch in diameter).

Cooking Instructions: Grill chicken breasts for 10 minutes on each side. Cube chicken. Combine peppers, vinegar, and mayonnaise in a blender. Put in a bowl and mix in the chicken. Add the spinach and mixture to tortilla.

Pasta Salad with Mixed Vegetables

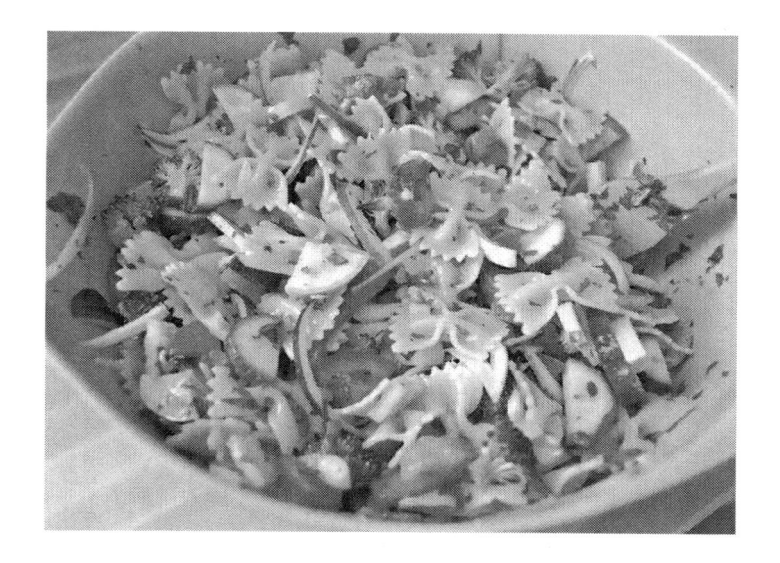

Serves: 8

Ingredients: 12 ounces whole-wheat rotini (spiral-shaped) pasta, 1 tablespoon olive oil, ¼ cup low-sodium chicken broth, 1 garlic clove, 2 medium onions (chopped), 1 can (28 ounces) unsalted chopped tomatoes in juice, 1 pound mushrooms, 1 red bell pepper (sliced), 1 green bell pepper (sliced), 2 medium zucchini (sliced), ½ teaspoon basil (shredded), ½ teaspoon oregano, 8 romaine lettuce leaves.

Cooking Instructions: Cook pasta according to the instructions on the container. Place in a large serving bowl, then add the olive oil and toss. Heat the chicken in a large skillet with the broth, adding the garlic, tomatoes, and onions for about five minutes. Add the herbs, then add the mixture to the pasta. Chill for an hour.

Soft Tacos with Southwestern Vegetables

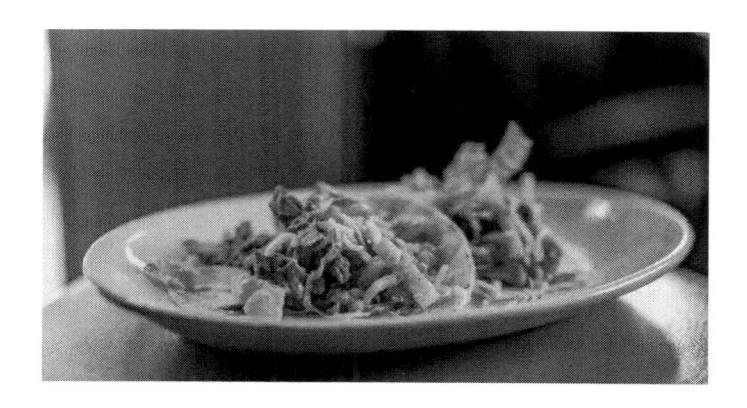

Serves: 4

Ingredients: 1 tablespoon olive oil, 1 medium red onion, 1 cup diced yellow summer squash, 1 cup diced green zucchini, 3 large garlic cloves, 4 medium tomatoes, seeded and chopped, 1 jalapeno chili (seeded and chopped), 1 cup fresh corn kernels (cut from about 2 ears of corn) or 1 cup frozen corn, 1 cup canned pinto or black beans (rinsed and drained), ½ cup chopped fresh cilantro, 8 corn tortillas, ½ cup smoke-flavored salsa.

Cooking Instructions: In a large pan, heat the olive oil over a medium heat. Add the onion and cook until tender, then add the spring squash and zucchini, and cook until tender, around 5 minutes. Mix in the garlic, tomatoes, jalapeno, corn and beans. Cook until the vegetables are tender, or around 5 minutes. Include the cilantro and remove from the high temperature. Heat a large pan (without a nonstick surface) over a medium heat. Place 1 tortilla in the hot dish and cook until browned— around 20 seconds for each side. Cook the remaining tortillas. To serve, place the tortillas on different plates. Scoop an equal portion of the vegetable mixture onto every tortilla. Add 2 tablespoons of the salsa to each plate.

Tuna Pita Pockets

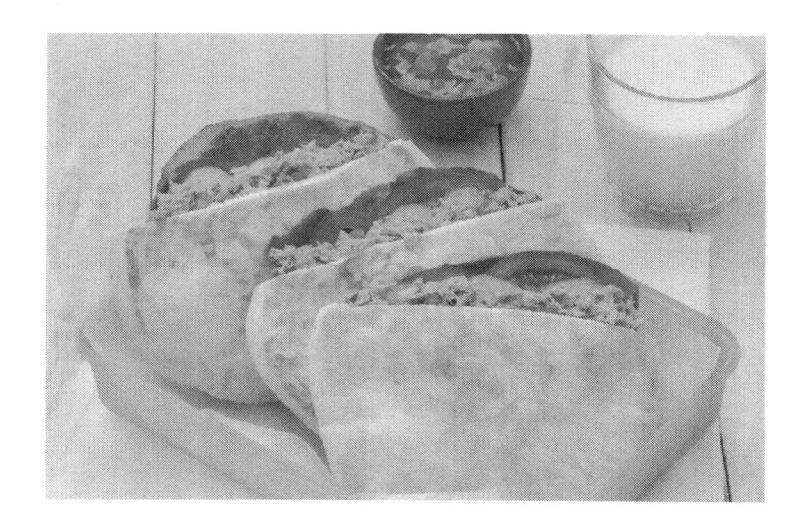

Serves: 6

Ingredients: 1½ cups shredded romaine lettuce, ¾ cup diced tomatoes, ½ cup finely chopped green bell peppers, ½ cup shredded carrots, ½ cup finely chopped broccoli, ¼ cup finely chopped onion, 2 cans (6 ounces each) low-salt white tuna (drained and packed in water), ½ cup low-fat ranch dressing, 3 whole-wheat pita pockets (cut into halves).

Cooking Instructions: In a large bowl, place the lettuce, tomatoes, peppers, carrots, broccoli and onions. In a small bowl, place the fish and dressing. Blend to mix well, then combine the tuna mixture and the lettuce mixture, then blend together.

Scoop ¾ cup of the tuna and mixed greens into every pita pocket half, then serve.

Salad Greens with Pears, Fennel and Walnuts

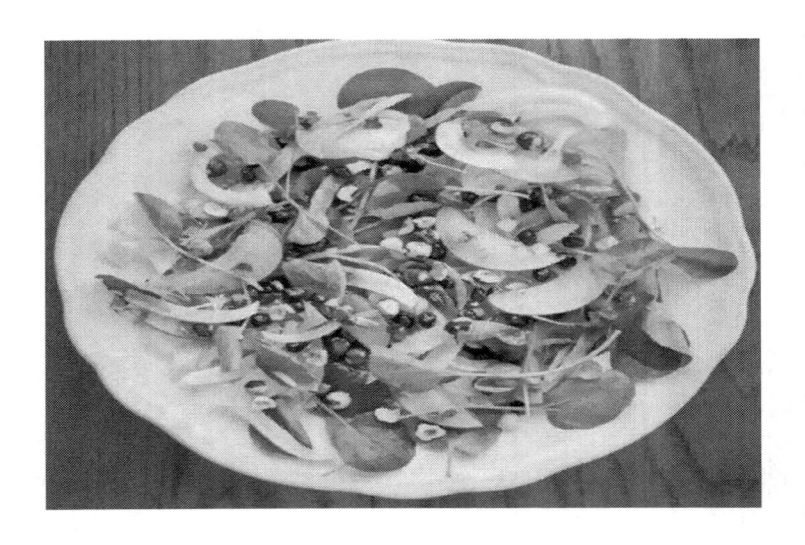

Serves: 6

Ingredients: 6 cups mixed salad greens, 1 medium fennel bulb, trimmed and thinly sliced, 2 medium pears (cored, quartered and thinly sliced), 2 tablespoons grated parmesan cheese, ¼ cup toasted and coarsely chopped walnuts, 3 tablespoons extra-virgin olive oil, 2 tablespoons balsamic vinegar, freshly-ground black pepper (to taste).

Cooking Instructions: Evenly distribute greens on six plates. Add the fennel and pear, then add the cheese and walnuts. Add the olive oil and vinegar then add pepper to taste.

Dinner Soups

Chicken Broth

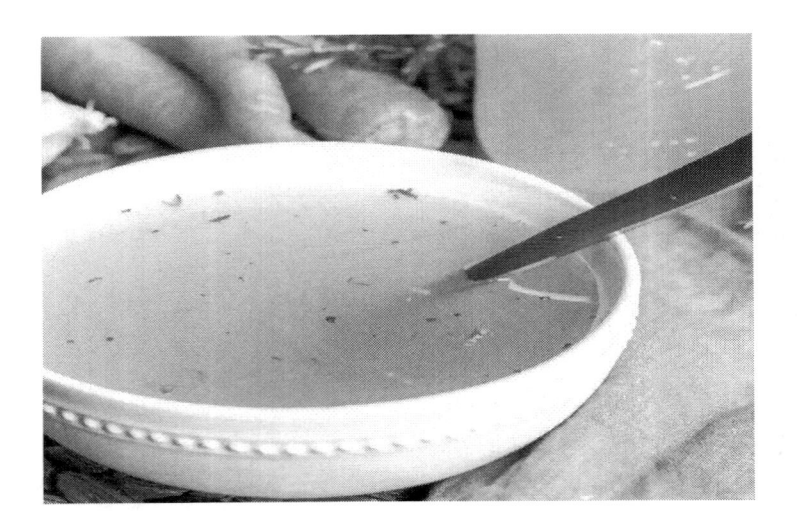

The slow cooker is perfect for making your own chicken broth. It is perfect for using as a base in your soups and other recipes.

Servings: 5

Ingredients: 2 pounds bone-in chicken pieces (any type will do), 6 cups water, 2 celery stalks (chopped), 2 medium carrots (chopped), 1 medium onion (chopped), 1 tablespoon basil (dried).

Cooking Instructions: Place all the ingredients into a slow cooker. Cover and cook on a low heat for 8 to 10 hours. Strain before using. Discard vegetables. Chicken can be used in soup or other recipe.

Nutritional Information (per serving): Calories 247, total fat 15 g, sodium 99mg, total carbohydratyes 6g, dietary fiber 1.8g, protein 22g.

Potato Leek Soup with Beans

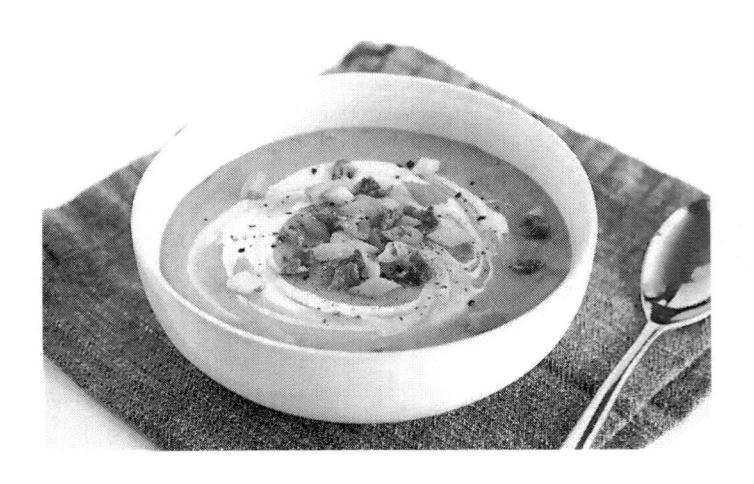

This soup is hearty enough to make a main dish.

Serves: 8

Ingredients: 2 leeks, ½ a medium white onion, 2 tbsps unsalted butter, 4 medium-sized potatoes (peeled and cubed), ½ parsnip (diced), 4 cups vegetable broth (low-sodium–homemade or store bought), 2 sprigs fresh rosemary, 2 sprigs fresh thyme, 1 can non-fat evaporated milk, 1 can white beans (cannellini or any other white bean with no-salt-added, drained and rinsed), freshly ground black pepper (to taste).

Cooking Instructions:

1. Slice the dark green tops off the leeks and the bottom roots off. You will be using only the white and light green parts of the leek, about 4-6 inches of leek. Rinse the leeks, then chop up into small slices. Dice the white onion. In a skillet, melt the unsalted butter over medium heat. Sauté the leek and onion for about 5 minutes, or until they begin to soften. Remove from heat and pour the leek, onion, and any melted butter still there into the slow cooker.
2. Add the potatoes, parsnip, broth, rosemary, thyme, evaporated milk, and white beans into the slow cooker. Stir properly.
3. Cover and cook on a low heat for 6-7 hours or on a high high for 4-5 hours, or until the potatoes and parsnip are soft.
4. Use and immersion blender to puree the soup to the desired consistency. Alternatively, transfer the contents to a blender or a large food processor, and puree it. (This may take two batches if your blender or processor is small.) Return the puree to the slow cooker and

heat it through for about 15 minutes. Season with pepper to taste. Serve hot.

Nutritional Information (per serving): Calorie: 251.9, total fat 3.4 g, sodium 109.2mg, total carbohydrates 44.1g, dietary fiber 6.4g, protein 11.2g.

Crockpot French Onion Soup

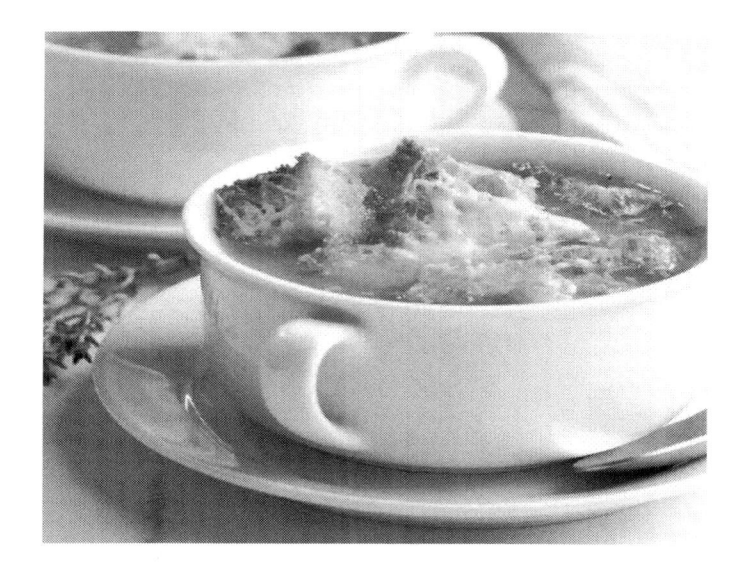

Serves: 8-10

Ingredients: 4 medium sweet onions (thinly sliced), 3 garlic cloves (minced), 4 tablespoons of unsalted butter, 2 tablespoons brown sugar, 2 tablespoons balsamic vinegar, 3 tablespoons all-purpose flour, 8 ounces of beer, 64 ounces of low-sodium beef stock, 2 tablespoons fresh thyme, ½ teaspoon black pepper, French bread, 8-10 pieces Gruyere cheese (sliced).

Cooking Instructions:

1. Heat a medium size skillet over medium heat. Add the onions, garlic, and butter, and sauté until the onions soften, for about 3-4 minutes. Add brown sugar and vinegar and mix until combined. Add to slow cooker.
2. Add in flour, beer, beef stock, thyme, and pepper. Stir, cover, and cook on low setting for 6-8 hours.
3. Before serving, Slice French bread into slices about an inch-thick. Fill oven-safe soup bowls with soup, top with slice of bread and a slice of cheese. Set under the broiler for 2-3 minutes, or until cheese is bubbly and golden brown. Serve at once.

Nutritional Information (per serving):
Calories 140, total fat 4.5g, sodium 505mg, total carbohydrates 19g, dietary fiber 2 g, protein 5 g.

Slow Cooker Chicken Noodle Soup

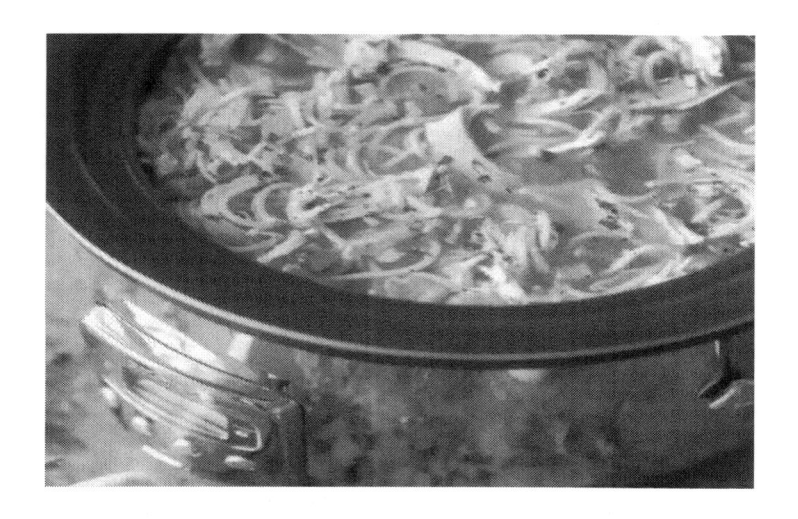

Nothing is more soothing than home-cooked chicken noodle soup.

Serves: 8

Ingredients: 2 pounds chicken (skinless and boneless, sliced into 2-inch pieces), 6 cups low-sodium chicken broth, ½ teaspoon crushed red pepper flakes, 1 cup celery (diced), 4 carrots (sliced), 1 small onion (diced), 3 cloves garlic (minced), ¼ cup fresh (chopped), Italian parsley, ½ teaspoon black pepper, a pinch of sea salt, 8 ounces whole wheat noodles.

Cooking Instructions:

1. Add all the ingredients, except the noodles, to the slow cooker and cook for 6-8 hours on a low heat, or until the carrots are tender.
2. In the last hour of cooking, add in the noodles and continue cooking for an additional hour, or until pasta is done to the desired effect.

Nutritional Information (per serving): Calories 149, total fat 2g, sodium 150mg, total carbohydrates 14g, dietary fiber 2g, protein 11g.

Hearty Minestrone Soup

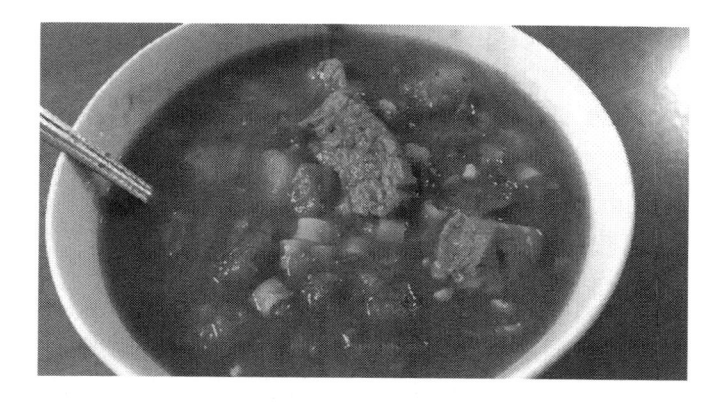

This soup provides a nice vegetarian dinner. Serve with some crusty whole-grain bread.

Serves: 8

Ingredients: 4 cups tomato juice (low-sodium), 4 cups vegetable broth (low-sodium), 1 medium onion (chopped), 4 cloves garlic (diced), 3 stalks celery (diced), 3 large carrots (sliced), 2 medium zucchini (chopped), 1 red pepper (diced), 1 15-ounce can white beans (rinsed and drained), 1 cup dried Stelline pasta (can substitute orzo, farfalline, or other small pasta), 2 teaspoons dried basil, 2 teaspoons dried oregano, freshly ground black pepper (to taste).

Cooking Instructions:

1. Place all the ingredients into a slow cooker. Cover, and cook on a low heat for 8-9 hours, or at a high heat for 4-5 hours, until the vegetables are tender.

Nutritional Information (per serving): calories 204, total fat 1g, sodium 180mg, total carbs 40g, protein 9g.

New England Clam Chowder

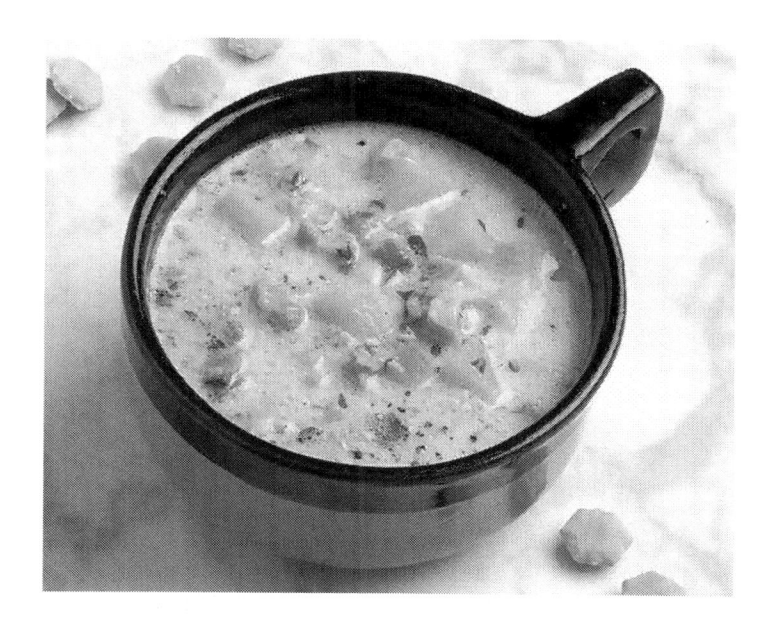

This hearty chowder is rich with potatoes and clams.

Serves: 10

Ingredients: 2 cups skim milk, 2 cups 1% milk, 2 unsalted tablespoons butter, 3 medium potatoes (peeled and diced), 1 medium yellow onion (chopped), 2 celery stalks (chopped), 1 bag of frozen sweet corn, 16 ounces of fresh clams in juice.

Cooking Instructions:

1. Place all ingredients into slow cooker.
2. Cover and cook for 2-3 hours on a high heat or 4-6 hours on a low heat. Onions should be soft and the potatoes should be tender.

Nutritional Information (per serving): calories 225.8, total fat 3.8g, sodium 112.7mg, total carbohydrates 34.1g, dietary fiber 2.4g, protein 5g.

Crock-Pot Lobster Bisque

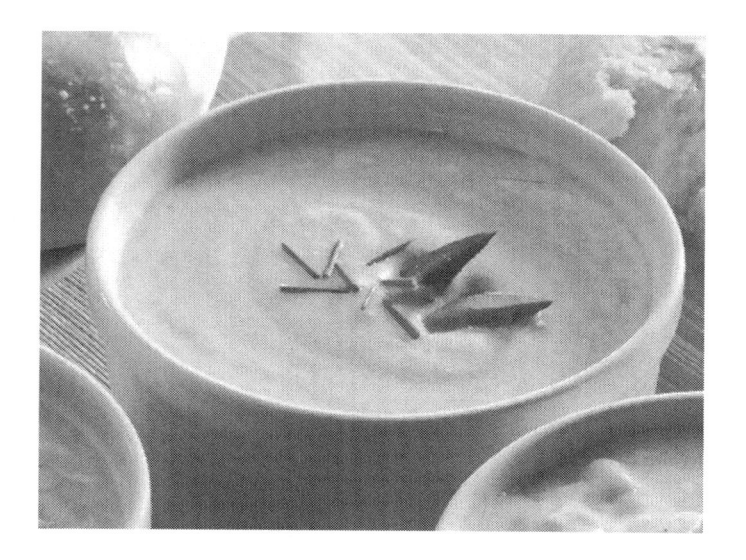

Serves: 6-8

Ingredients: 1 teaspoon olive oil, 2 shallots (minced), 1 clove garlic (minced), 2 14.5-ounce cans diced tomatoes (no salt added), 1 32-ounce carton low-sodium chicken broth (or homemade), 1 tablespoon Old Bay seasoning, 1 teaspoon dried dill, ¼ cup fresh parsley (chopped), 1 teaspoon freshly ground black pepper, ½ teaspoon paprika, 3 lobster tails, 1 pint heavy cream.

Cooking Instructions:

1. Heat olive oil in skillet over medium heat. Add shallots and garlic, then sauté for 2-3 minutes. Add shallot and garlic mixture to slow cooker.
2. Add tomatoes, chicken broth, Old Bay seasoning, dill, parsley, pepper, and paprika to slow cooker.
3. Using a sharp knife, slice off the fan part of the end of the lobsters and add those to a slow cooker, reserving the lobster tails for later.
4. Stir, cover, and cook on a low heat for 6 hours, or a high heat for 3 hours.
5. Remove the lobster tail ends from the cooker and discard.
6. Using an immersion blender, puree the soup mixture to the desired effect. You can also use a regular blender, in batches.
7. Add the lobster tails to the soup, cover, and cook for about an hour on a low heat, or until the shells turn red and the lobster meat is cooked.
8. Remove the lobster tails from the soup and let them cool slightly. Slice each lobster tail in half length-ways and remove the lobster flesh from the shells.

Discard the shells and roughly chop the lobster meat and add it back into the soup.
9. Add the cream and stir.

Nutritional Information (per serving): calories 380, total fat 27g, sodium 330mg, total carbs 15g, dietary fiber, 1g protein 22g.

Meatball Soup

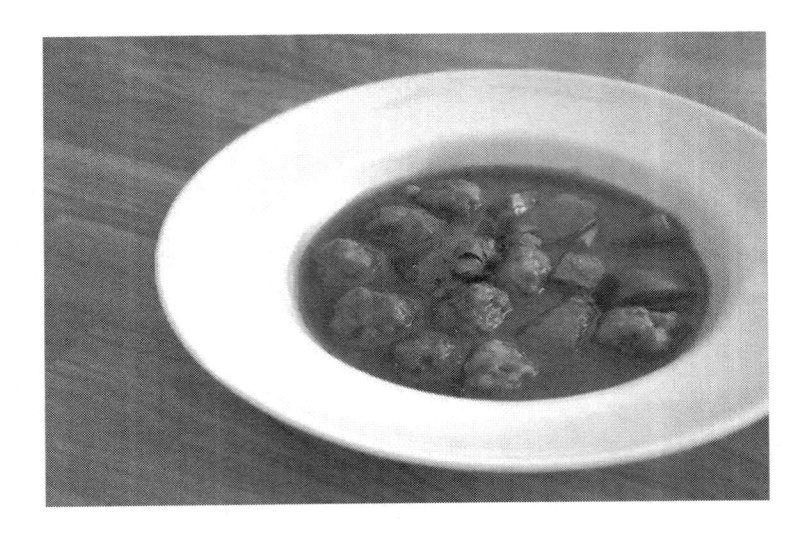

This hearty soup is perfect on a cold winter day.

Serves: 6

Ingredients: For the meatballs: 1 pound ground beef (lean 90/10), ½ pound ground pork, ¼ cup bread crumbs, 3 garlic cloves (minced), 1 small yellow onion (finely chopped), 1 egg (beaten), 1 tablespoon Italian seasoning, 1 teaspoon black pepper, 2 tablespoons olive oil. For the soup: 4 slices bacon (sliced into pieces), 3 cloves garlic (minced), 1 medium zucchini (chopped), 1 medium yellow squash (chopped), 2 carrots (sliced thin), 1 small onion (finely diced) 1 teaspoon oregan, 1 teaspoon marjora, 1 teaspoon garlic powder, 4 cups chicken broth (low sodium), 1 14.5-ounce can diced tomatoes (no salt added).

Cooking Instructions:

1. In a large bowl, mix together all ingredients for meatballs except for the olive oil. Form into balls about 1½ to 2 inches in diameter.
2. Heat olive oil in large skillet over a medium heat. Add the meatballs and cook until all sides are browned. Remove the meatballs and set aside. Add the bacon to pan and sauté for 4-5 minutes. Add the garlic and sauté for another 2 minutes.
3. Place the bacon and garlic (along with drippings) into a slow cooker. Place the meatballs on top.
4. Add in all remaining ingredients. Stir gently to mix.
5. Cover and cook on a low heat for 8 hours or on a high heat for 5 hours.

Nutritional Information (per serving): calories 295, total fat 17g, sodium 195mg, total carbs 11g, protein 21g.

Chicken Tortilla Soup

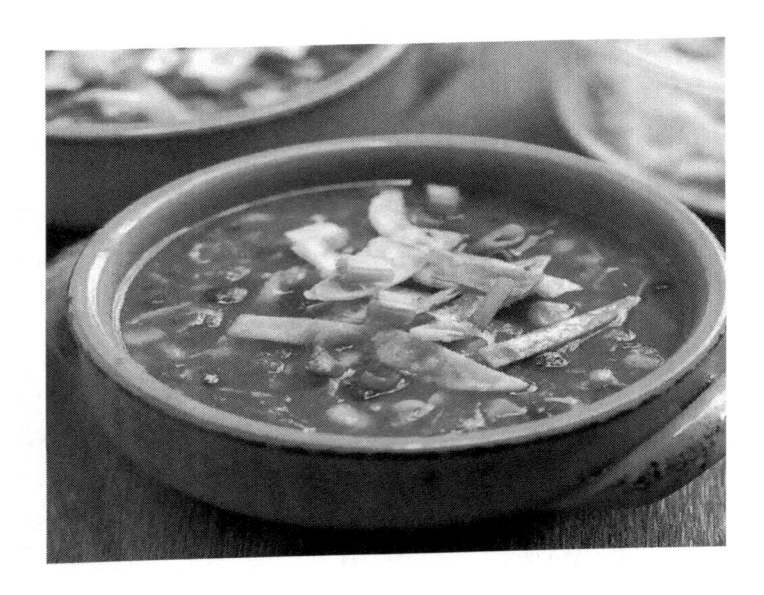

This is a healthier, low-sodium version of a popular soup.

Serves: 8

Ingredients: 1 pound chicken, boneless and skinless (sliced into bite-size pieces), 1 15-ounce can whole tomatoes (mashed) 1 10-ounce can enchilada sauce, 1 medium onion (chopped), 2 chili peppers (chopped), 3 cloves garlic (minced), 2 cups water, 2 cups low-sodium chicken broth, 1 10-ounce package frozen corn, 2 teaspoons cumin, 2 teaspoons chili powder, ½ teaspoon salt, ½ teaspoon freshly ground black pepper, 1 bay leaf, 1 tablespoon fresh cilantro (chopped), 8 corn tortillas.

Cooking Instructions:

1. Place the chicken, tomatoes, enchilada sauce, onion, pepper, and garlic into a slow cooker. Add in the water, chicken broth and corn. Season with cumin, chili powder, salt, pepper, bay leaf, and cilantro.
2. Cover and cook on a low heat for 7-8 hours, or a high heat for 3-4 hours.
3. Slice tortillas into strips. Place on a baking sheet and cook in a preheated 400°F oven for about 10 minutes until crisp.
4. Serve soup with tortilla strips sprinkled on top. It may also be topped with fresh avocado slices, shredded cheese, or fresh cilantro.

Nutritional Information (per serving): Calories 210, total fat 6.8g, sodium 398mg, total carbohydrates 24g, dietary fiber 3.9 g, protein 15g.

Corn and Shrimp Chowder

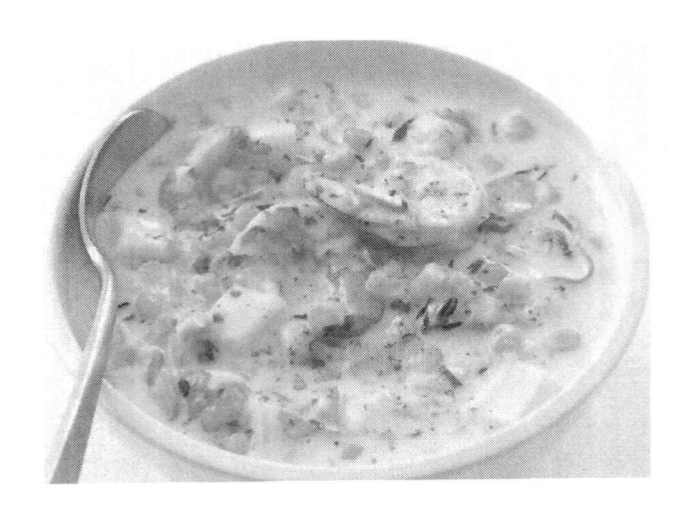

Most recipes for corn and shrimp chowder have too much sodium for the DASH diet. Here we have reduced the sodium without reducing the flavor.

Serves: 6

Ingredients: 3 cups chicken broth (low-sodium), 2 cups water, 2 16-ounce bags frozen corn, 1 medium yellow onion (chopped), 2 large carrots (chopped), 1 red bell pepper (chopped), 3 medium potatoes (diced), 2 bay leaves, 2 teaspoon Old Bay seasoning, 1 teaspoon cayenne pepper, 1 pound medium shrimp (peeled) ½ cup whole milk, ⅓ cup fresh parsley, freshly ground black pepper (to taste).

Cooking Instructions:

1. Add the chicken broth, water, corn, onion, carrots, pepper, potatoes, bay leaves, Old Bay, and cayenne pepper to a slow cooker. Cover and cook on a low heat for 5-6 hours, or until the vegetables are tender.
2. Using an immersion blender, puree soup until desired consistency is reached. Alternatively, in batches, blend soup in a traditional blender until desired consistency is reached and return to slow cooker.
3. Add shrimp and milk, stir, cover, and cook for another 15 minutes until shrimp is pink.
4. Remove bay leaves, sprinkle with parsley, and season with black pepper before serving.

Nutritional Information (per serving): Calories 550, total fat 6g, sodium 391mg, total carbohydrates 97g, dietary fiber 6g, protein 31g.

Split Pea Soup

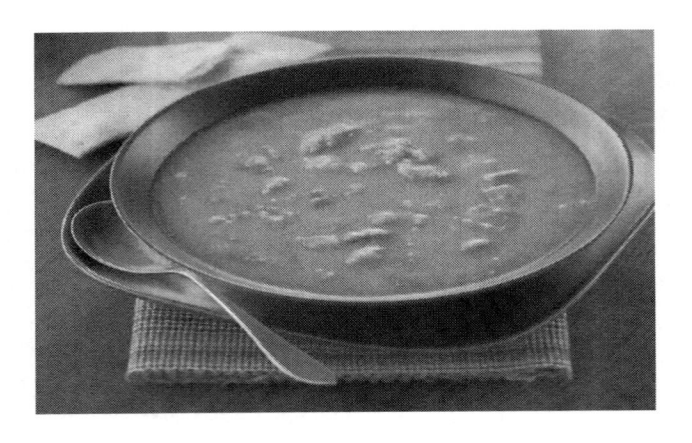

This classic soup works properly in a slow cooker.

Serves: 6

Ingredients: 7 cups chicken broth (low-sodium), 1 bag green or yellow split peas (rinsed and drained), 1 medium onion (diced), 4 carrots (diced), 1 celery stalk (diced) ½ red bell pepper (diced), 3 cloves garlic (minced), 1 teaspoon dried thyme, 1 bay leaf, 1 ham hock, freshly ground black pepper (to taste).

Cooking Instructions:

1. Add all ingredients to a slow cooker. Stir, cover, and cook on high for 6-7 hours or until split peas are creamy.

2. Remove ham hocks. Remove and discard skin and bones. Dice meat and return to slow cooker. Remove bay leaf before serving.

Nutritional Information (per serving): Calories 370, sodium 180mg, protein 28g, Carbohydrates 62g, dietary fiber 25g, fat 3.5g.

Poultry Dishes

Mexican Chicken Stew

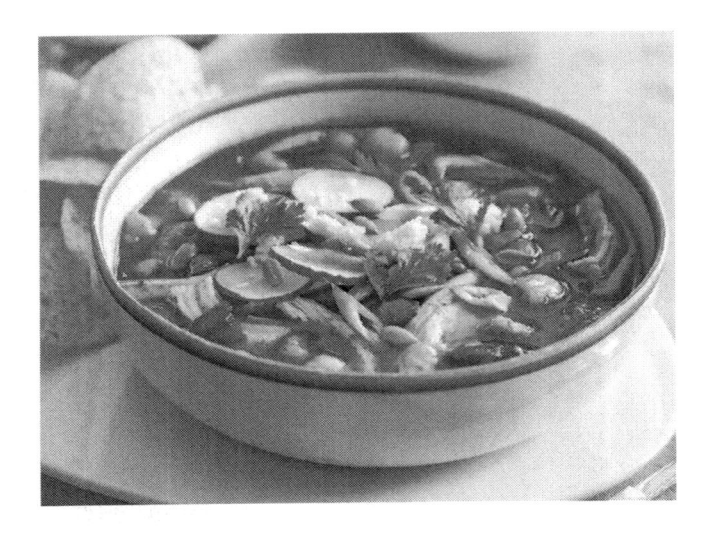

This spicy stew is very easy to prepare.

Serves: 12

Ingredients: 4 chicken breasts (boneless and skinless), 1 15.5-ounce can whole kernel corn (no-salt added), 1 15.5-ounce can kidney beans (no-sodium added) 1 15.5-ounce can black beans (no-sodium added) 1 15.5-ounce can diced tomatoes (no-salt added) 1 medium yellow onion (diced), 1 green bell pepper (diced), 1 15.5-ounce can tomato sauce (no-salt added), 2 tablespoons chili powder, 2 teaspoons onion powder, 2 teaspoons ground cumin, 1 teaspoon garlic powder • 1 teaspoon paprika, 1 teaspoon ground oregano.

Cooking Instructions:

1. Place the chicken breasts in slow cooker. Add the remaining ingredients, and stir gently, leaving the chicken on the bottom.
2. Cover and cook on a high heat for 3-4 hours or a low heat for 5-6 hours. Remove the chicken breasts and shred or chop them, then add back to the stew. Mix properly before serving.

Nutritional Information (per serving): Calories 208.5, total fat 1.6g, sodium 162.3mg, carbohydrates 23.3g, dietary fiber 5.9g, protein 25.6g.

Crockpot Chicken Fajitas

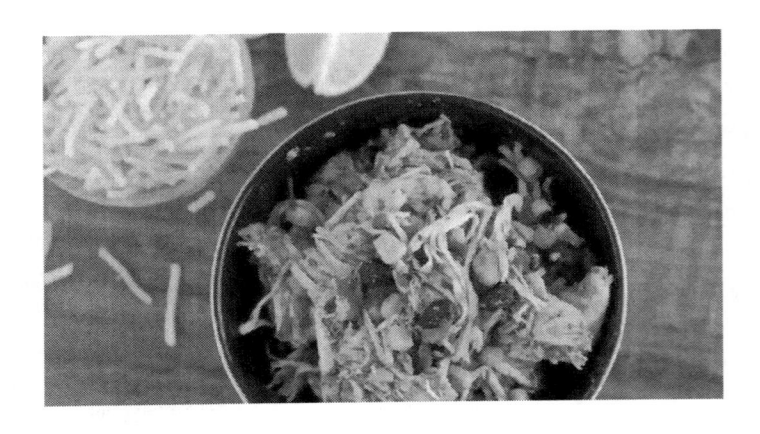

Serves: 4

Ingredients: 1 pound chicken breast (boneless and skinless), 1 medium onion (sliced into strips), 1 medium red bell pepper (sliced into strips), 1 medium green bell pepper (sliced into strips), 3 garlic cloves (minced), 1 tablespoon taco seasoning, 1 cup salsa.

Cooking Instructions:

1. Place the chicken breast in a crockpot. Slice the onion, peppers, and garlic, and place on top of chicken. Top with salsa. Cover and cook for 7-8 hours on a low heat or 5-6 hours on a high heat.
2. Shred chicken and serve with tortillas.

Nutritional Information (per serving): Calories 176.0, total fat 1.6g, sodium 156.2mg, total carbs 11.3g, dietary fiber 1.6g, protein 27.2g.

Black Bean Chicken

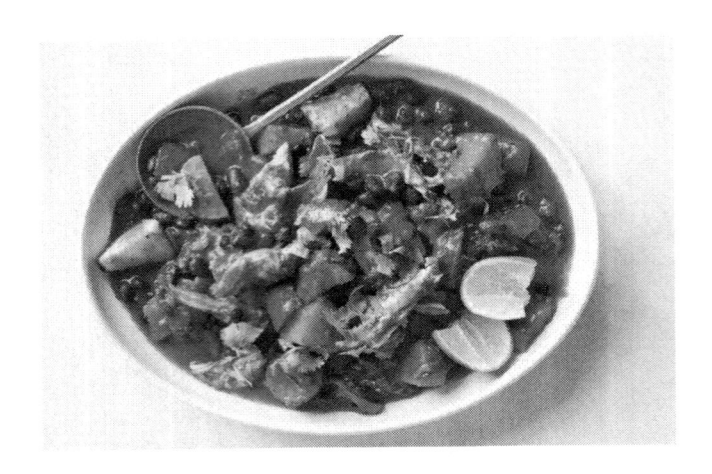

This is a very simple recipe but it is very tasty.

Serves: 6

Ingredients: 1 pound boneless skinless chicken breasts, 2 15-ounce cans black beans (low-sodium, rinsed and drained), 2 cups salsa (if buying jarred, make sure it is low in sodium), ½ cup brown rice (uncooked).

Cooking Instructions: Place the chicken breasts in a slow cooker. Pour the beans, rice, and salsa over the chicken, and stir to combine. Cover and cook on a low heat for 8-10 hours. Serve hot.

Nutritional Information (per serving): Calories 307.3, total fat 2.9g, sodium 146.4mg, total carbohydrates 40.0g, dietary fiber 13.0g, protein 30g.

Turkey Chili

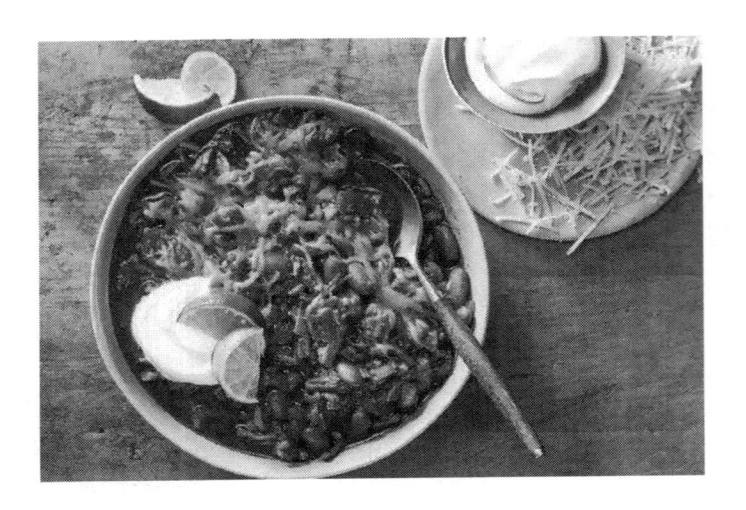

Serves: 8

Ingredients: 1 tablespoon olive oil, 1 pound ground turkey, 2 10.75-ounce cans tomato soup (low-sodium), 2 15-ounce cans red kidney beans (low-sodium, rinsed and drained), 1 15-ounce can black beans (drained), ½ medium onion (chopped), 2 tablespoons chili powder, 1 teaspoon red pepper flakes, ½ tablespoon garlic powder, ½ tablespoon ground cumin, freshly ground black pepper (to taste), ½ teaspoon ground allspice.

Cooking Instructions:

1. Heat the oil in a skillet over medium heat. Add the ground turkey to the skillet, and cook until browned, then drain.
2. Spray slow cooker with cooking spray, and add turkey, tomato soup, kidney beans, black beans, and onion. Season with chili powder, red pepper flakes, garlic powder, cumin, black pepper, allspice, and salt.
3. Cover and cook for 7-8 hours on a low heat, or 4-5 hours on a high heat.

Nutritional Information (per serving):
Calories 520, total fat 8g, sodium 390mg, total carbs 14g, dietary fiber 21g, protein 38g.

Mediterranean Roast Turkey Breast

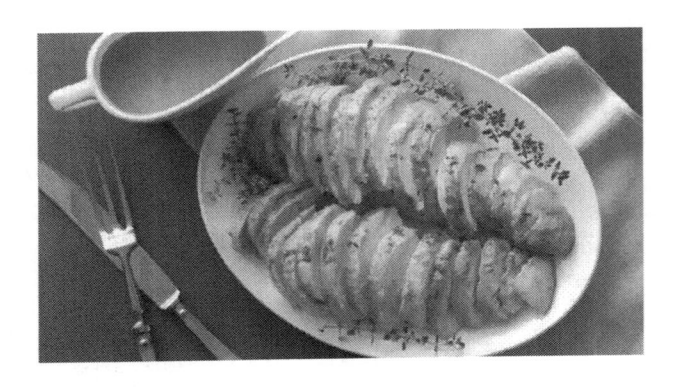

This Mediterranean-inspired dish is full-flavored and aromatic.

Serves: 8

Ingredients: 1 boneless turkey breast (about 3½-4 pounds), 1 cup chicken broth (low-sodium) 2 tablespoons lemon juice, 2 medium yellow onions (chopped) ½ cup kalamata olives (pitted), 1 teaspoon garlic powder, 1 teaspoon basil, 1 teaspoon oregano, ½ teaspoon cinnamon, ½ teaspoon rosemary, ½ teaspoon freshly ground black pepper, 1 12-ounce jar artichoke hearts, ½ cup sun-dried tomatoes (oil-packed, sliced).

Cooking Instructions:

1. Place the turkey breast in a slow cooker. Add the chicken broth, lemon juice, onions, olives, and spices. Stir, cover, and cook on a low heat for 6 hours.
2. Add in artichoke hearts and sun-dried tomatoes. Stir, cover, and cook for an additional 30 minutes to an hour.
3. Serve over brown rice.

Nutritional Information (per serving):
Calories 356, total fat 4.8g, sodium 365mg, total carbs 9g, dietary fiber 1.6g, protein 60g.

Honey-Glazed Chicken Wings

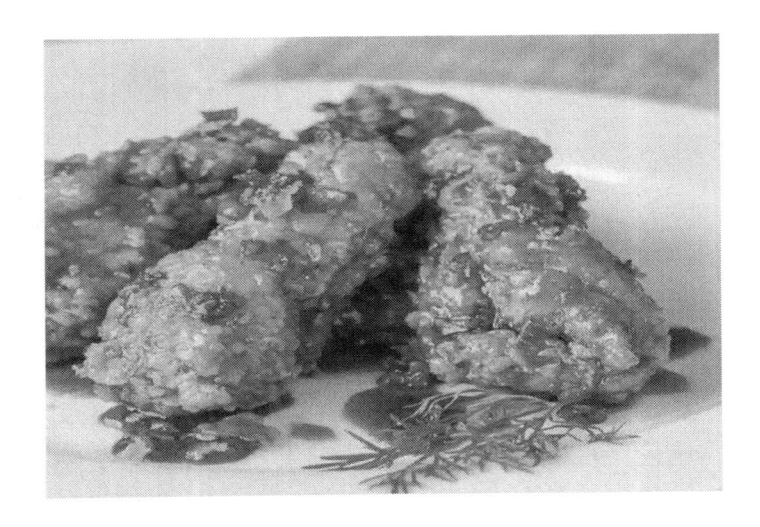

These wings are spicy and sweet.

Serves: 8

Ingredients: ½ cup rice wine vinegar, 5 tablespoons honey, 3 tablespoons soy sauce (low-sodium), ¼ cup sesame oil, 2 tablespoons lemon juice, 3 tablespoons Asian chili paste, 5 cloves garlic, minced, 1 tablespoon freshly grated ginger (or ½ teaspoon dried ginger), freshly ground black pepper (to taste), 2 pounds chicken wings, 2 tablespoons toasted sesame seeds.

Cooking Instructions:

1. In a bowl, whisk together all the ingredients except for chicken wings and sesame seeds.
2. Place the chicken wings in a slow cooker. Pour sauce over the wings and stir to coat chicken.
3. Cover and cook on a low heat for 4-5 hours, or a high heat for 2-3 hours, until chicken is cooked through.
4. Serve sprinkled with toasted sesame seeds.

Nutritional Information (per serving): Calories 321, total fat 19g, sodium 428mg, total carbs 14g, protein 22g.

Jambalaya

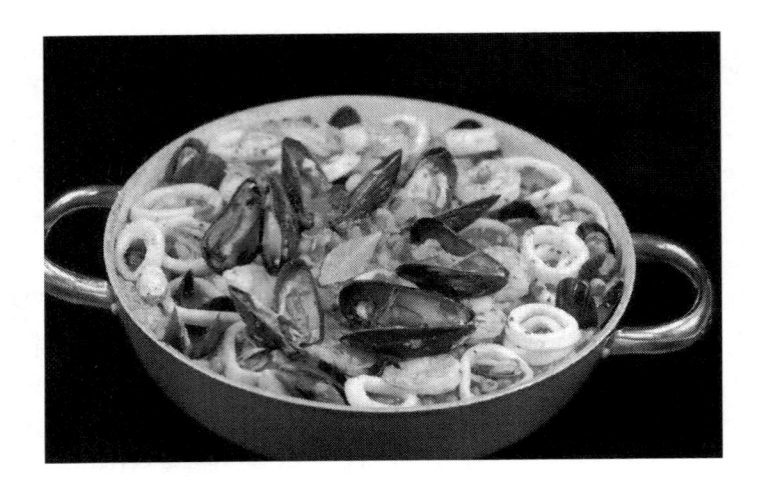

This is a spicy Cajun dish reformulated to cut the sodium down without compromising the flavor.

Serves: 6

Ingredients: 1 pound chicken breast, skinless and boneless, Slice into 1-2 inch chunks, ½ pound andouille sausage (crumbled), 2 15-ounce cans of chopped tomatoes (no salt added), 1 large green bell pepper (chopped), 1 medium yellow onion (chopped), 1 cup chicken broth (low-sodium), ½ cup white wine, 2 teaspoons oregano, 1 tablespoon fresh parsle, 2 teaspoon Cajun seasoning, 1 teaspoon cayenne pepper, ½ pound medium shrimp (peeled), 2 cups cooked brown rice.

Cooking Instructions:

1. Place all ingredients except for the shrimps and rice in a slow cooker. Stir, cover and cook on a low heat for 6-8 hours, or on a high heat for 3-4 hours.
2. Add in the shrimp and rice. Cover and cook for an additional 30 minutes.

Nutritional Information (per serving): Calories 430, total fat 18g, sodium 188mg, total carbs 23g, dietary fiber 2g, protein 40g.

Slow-Cooker Turkey Stroganoff

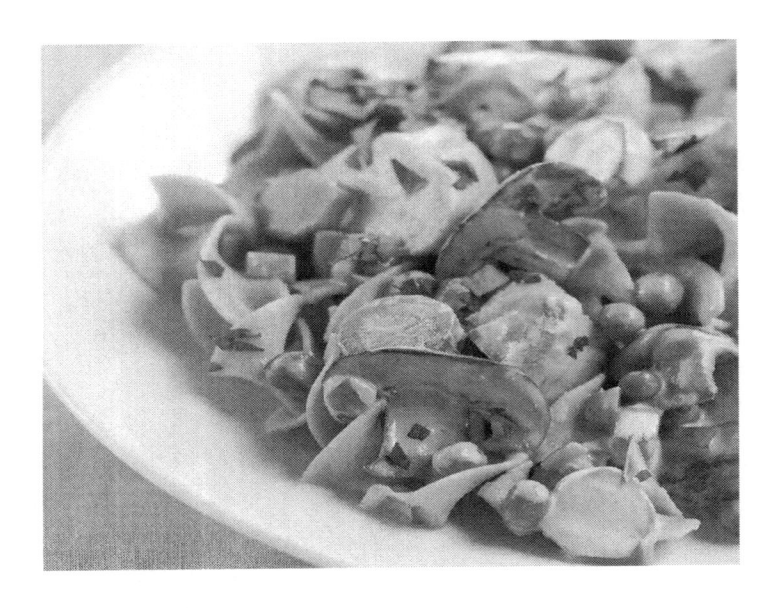

Serves: 6

Ingredients: 4 cups mushrooms(sliced–can use a mix of types), 3 medium carrots (sliced), 1 small onion (diced), 1 3-4 pound split turkey breast (skin removed–can substitute with a chicken breast), ⅓ cup all-purpose flour, 1 cup non-fat Greek-style plain yogurt, 1 tablespoon lemon juice, ¼ cup dry sherry (not cooking sherry), 1 cup frozen peas (thawed) freshly ground black pepper (to taste), 12 ounces whole-wheat egg noodles (cooked), ¼ cup flat-leaf parsley (chopped).

Cooking Instructions:

1. Place mushrooms, carrots, onion, and turkey into a slow cooker. Cover and cook on a low heat for 8 hours, or on a high heat for 4 hours.
2. Remove the turkey from the slow cooker and slice meat from the bone. Slice into bite size pieces and put back in the slow cooker.
3. In a bowl, whisk together flour, yogurt, lemon juice, and sherry. Add to the slow cooker along with the peas and pepper. Stir, cover, and cook on high for another 20 minutes.
4. Serve over egg noodles and top with chopped parsley.

Nutritional Information (per serving): Calories 440, sodium 480mg, protein 46g, carbohydrates 43g, fat 6g.

Provencal Chicken and White Beans

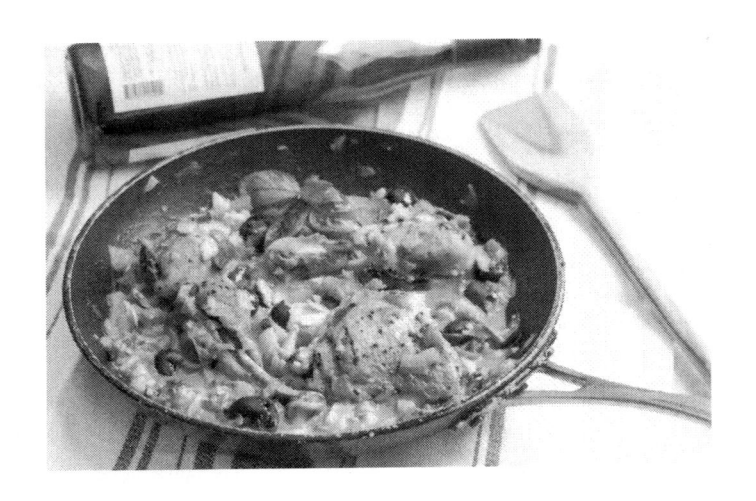

Another very easy recipe that tastes like you spent a lot of time in the kitchen.

Serves: 6

Ingredients: 1½ pounds chicken breast (boneless and skinless), 1 red bell pepper (diced), 1 16-ounce can cannellini beans (low sodium–rinsed and drained), 1 14.5-ounce can diced tomatoes (no salt added), ¼ teaspoon salt, ½ teaspoon freshly ground black pepper, 2 teaspoon basil, 2 teaspoon oregano, 1 teaspoon thyme.

Cooking Instructions:

1. Place all ingredients in a slow cooker. Stir, cover, and cook on low for 7-8 hours.

Nutritional Information (per serving): Calories 225, sodium 489mg, protein 29g, carbs 20g, fat 3g.

White Chicken Chili

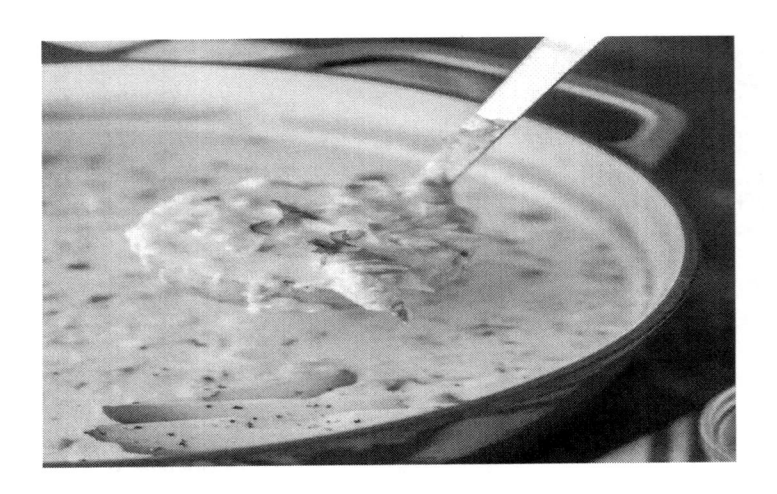

Serves: 6

Ingredients: 2 15-ounce cans white beans (Great Northern or cannellini, no-salt added), 1 pound chicken (boneless and skinless, sliced into chunks), 1 15-ounce can diced tomatoes (no salt added), 1 4.5-ounce can green chilies (drained and chopped), 1 medium yellow onion (chopped), 3 cloves garlic (minced), 1 tablespoon chili powder, 1 teaspoon cumin, 1 teaspoon oregano, 1 teaspoon cayenne pepper.

Cooking Instructions:

1. Add all ingredients to a slow cooker. Stir to combine, cover and cook on low for 8 hours or high for 4 hours.

Nutritional Information (per serving): Calories 285, sodium 260mg, protein 25g, carbs 34g, dietary fiber 8g, fat 5.7g.

Desserts

Slow Cooker Brown Rice Pudding

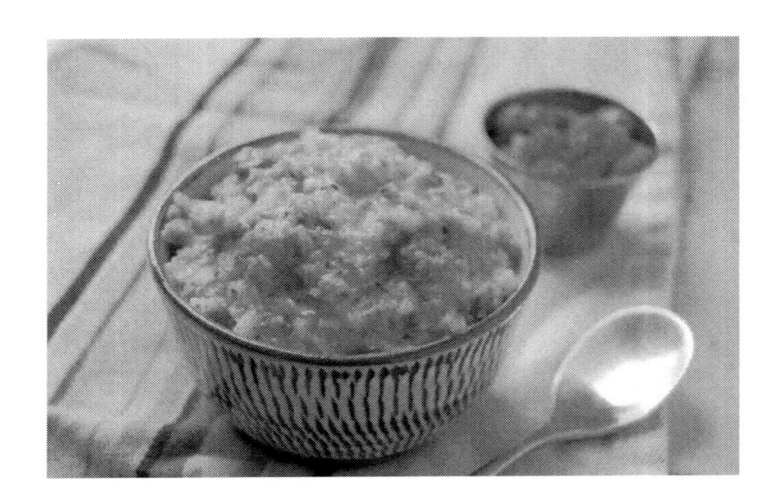

Serves: 6

Ingredients: ⅔ cup brown rice (long grain), 1 teaspoon cinnamon, ¼ cup honey, 1 ⅔ cups milk (low-fat), 1 13.5-ounce can coconut milk (low-fat), 1 teaspoon vanilla extract, ½ cup raisins (optional).

Cooking Instructions:

1. Add all ingredients except the vanilla and raisins to a slow cooker. Stir to combine. Cover and cook on a low heat

for 3-4 hours until desired consistency is reached.
2. Add the vanilla and raisins, stir, cover the slow cooker and turn off. Let sit for 15 minutes before serving.

Nutritional Information (per serving): Calories 245, total fat 14g, sodium 50mg, total carbohydrates 29g, dietary fiber 1g, protein 4g.

Berry Cobbler

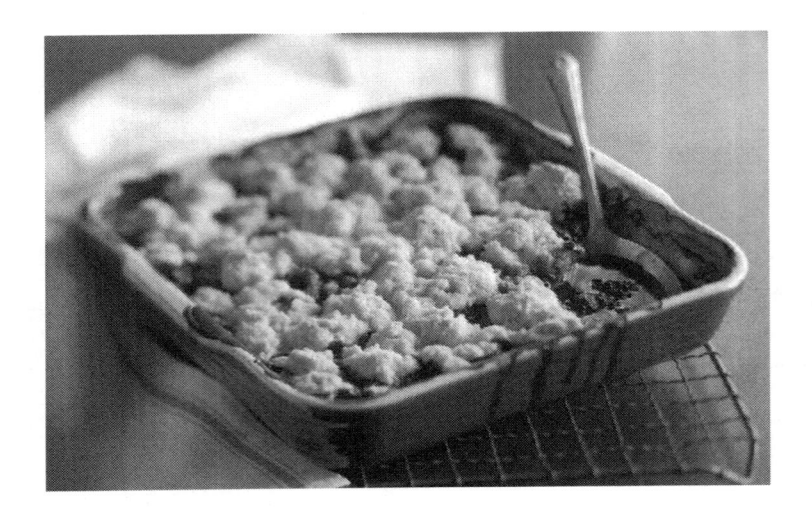

Serves: 8

Ingredients: 1¼ cups all-purpose flour, divided, 1 cup sugar plus 2 tablespoons, divided, 1 teaspoon baking powder, ½ teaspoon cinnamon, 1 egg (beaten), ¼ cup skim milk, 2 tablespoons olive oil, ⅛ teaspoon salt, 2 cups raspberries (fresh or frozen, thawed), 2 cups blueberries (fresh or frozen, thawed), vanilla yogurt for topping (optional).

Cooking Instructions:

1. Combine 1 cup flour, 2 tablespoons sugar, baking powder and cinnamon in a large bowl.

2. In a separate bowl, mix together the egg, milk, and oil. Fold in dry ingredients until just moistened (batter will be thick).
3. Spray bottom of slow cooker with nonstick spray. Spread batter evenly into bottom of slow cooker.
4. In a large bowl, combine the salt and remaining flour and sugar, add the berries and toss to coat. Spread over batter.
5. Cover and cook on high for 2 to 2½ hours, or until a toothpick inserted into the cobbler comes out clean.
6. Serve topped with yogurt.

Nutritional Information (per serving): Calories 250, total fat 4g, sodium 140mg total carbs 51g, dietary fiber 4g, protein 3g.

Spiced Apple Sauce

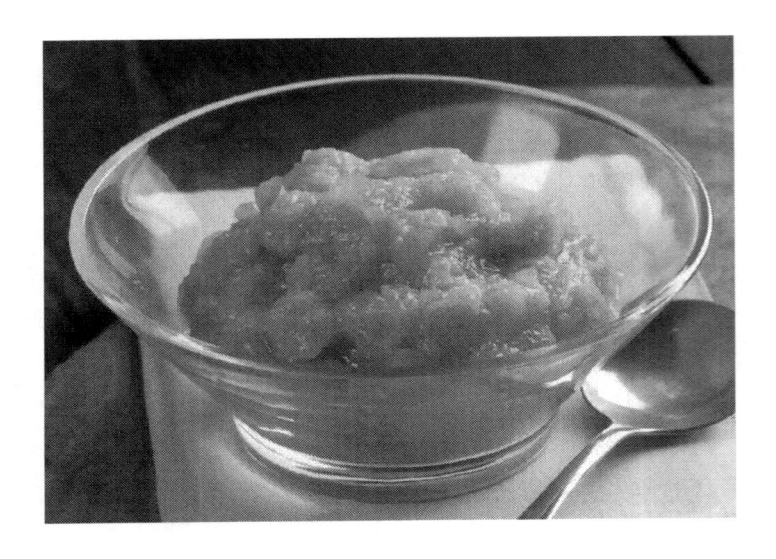

This apple sauce is easy and makes a nice, warm, healthy treat on a cold day.

Serves: 8

Ingredients: 8 apples (peeled, cored, and sliced–can use a combination, Granny Smith, Gala, Golden Delicious, etc.), ⅓ cup water, ⅓ cup brown sugar (packed), ½ teaspoon pumpkin pie spice, ¼ teaspoon nutmeg.

Cooking Instructions:

1. Combine all the ingredients in a slow cooker. Stir, cover and cook on a low heat for 6 to 8 hours.

Nutritional Information (per serving): Calories 98, total fat 0.2g, sodium 3mg, total carbohydrates 26g, dietary fiber 1.7g protein .4 g.

Apple Crisp

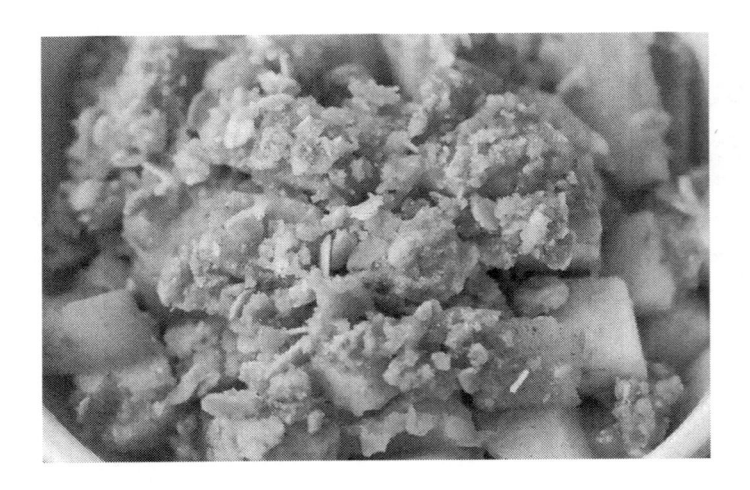

Really delicious and super easy in the slow cooker.

Serves: 6

Ingredients: 1 cup all-purpose flour, ½ cup oats, ½ cup brown sugar (packed), ⅔ cup white sugar (divided), 1½ teaspoon cinnamon (divided), ½ teaspoon nutmeg, pinch of salt, 4 tablespoons butter (slice into pieces), 1 cup walnuts (chopped), 1 tablespoon cornstarch, 1 teaspoon ginger, 6 cups apples (about 6-7 large apples, peeled, cored, and cubed), 2 tablespoons lemon juice.

Cooking Instructions:

1. In a bowl, mix together flour, oats, brown sugar, ⅓ cup white sugar, 1 teaspoon cinnamon, nutmeg, and salt. Add in the butter pieces and use your hands or a fork to mix together until crumbs form. Stir in the walnuts.
2. In a separate bowl, mix together ⅓ cup sugar, cornstarch, ginger, and ½ teaspoon cinnamon.
3. Place apples in slow cooker. Stir in the sugar and cornstarch mixture. Sprinkle on lemon juice and stir. Sprinkle butter and walnut mixture evenly on the top. Cover and cook on a low heat for 3-4 hours or a high heat for 2 hours, or until the apples are tender.

Nutritional Information (per serving): Calories 565, total fat 29g, sodium 118mg, total carbohydrates 84g, dietary fiber 6g, protein 6g.

Meat Dishes (Beef, Pork, Lamb, Veal)

Barbecued Pork

Serves: 6-8

Ingredients: ½ pound pork (slicelets, boneless), 1 cup celery (chopped), 1 medium onion (chopped), 2 cloves garlic (minced), 1 teaspoon olive oil, 1 6-ounce can tomato paste (no salt added), 1 8-ounce can tomato sauce (no salt added), 2 tablespoons white vinegar, 1 teaspoon Worcestershire sauce, 2 teaspoons chopped parsley, ¼ teaspoon pepper, ½ teaspoon garlic powder, 1 tablespoon packed brown sugar, 1 teaspoon chili powder.

Cooking Instructions:

1. Slice pork slicelets into 1-2 inch cubes.
2. Heat the olive oil in large skillet over a medium heat. Add the pork cubes and brown on all sides, for about 4-5 minutes. Place in a slow cooker. Add celery, onion, and garlic to a skillet and sauté until they begin to soften, or around 2-3 minutes. Add to a slow cooker with pork.

3. In a bowl, combine sauce ingredients (tomato paste through chili powder), and then pour into a slow cooker over pork and vegetables. Stir to combine.
4. Cover and cook on a low heat for 7-8 hours, or a high heat for 5-6 hours.

Nutritional Information (per serving): Calories 335, total fat 13.5g, sodium 115mg, total carbs 9.9g, dietary fiber 1.4g, protein 42.7g.

Slow Cooker Chili

Serves: 11 (1 cup servings)

Ingredients: 1 cup dry pinto beans, 1 cup dry dark red kidney beans, 1 cup light red kidney beans, 1 cup water, ½ pound ground turkey, ½ pound lean ground beef, 3 medium yellow onions (chopped), 1 large green bell pepper (chopped), 1 large red bell pepper (chopped), 3 cloves garlic (minced), 6 large tomatoes (chopped), 1 teaspoon cayenne pepper, 1 tablespoon cumin, ½ tablespoon marjoram, 1 teaspoon freshly ground black pepper 1 tablespoon chili powder, 1 tablespoon oregano.

Cooking Instructions:

1. Place beans in large bowl, cover with water, and soak overnight. Rinse and drain properly.
2. Heat a large skillet over medium heat. Add the ground beef and ground turkey and cook until browned. Add browned meat to a slow cooker. In same pan, sauté onions, pepper, and garlic until just softened, for about 3-4 minutes. Add to the slow cooker.

3. Add soaked and drained beans, chopped tomatoes, and spices to the slow cooker. Stir properly.
4. Cover and cook for 7-8 hours on a low heat.

Nutritional Information (per serving): Calories 181.8, total fat 3.5g, sodium 63mg, total carbs 33g, dietary fiber 15g, protein 18.4g.

Spaghetti Sauce with Meat and Vegetables

Jarred sauce typically has a large amount of sodium. Make your own without salt and include some extra vegetables too.

Serves: 6-8

Ingredients: ½ pound ground turkey, ½ pound ground beef (lean), 1 large yellow onion (diced fine), 3 cloves garlic (minced), 1 green pepper (diced fine), 1 medium zucchini (diced), 1 medium yellow/crookneck squash (diced), 1 pound sliced mushrooms, 1 6-ounce can tomato paste (no salt added), 6 large tomatoes (diced), 1 cup red wine, 1 tablespoon garlic powder, 1 tablespoon oregano, ½ tablespoon dried basil, 1 tablespoon Italian seasoning, freshly ground black pepper, to taste.

Cooking Instructions:

1. Heat a large nonstick skillet over a medium heat. Add the ground turkey and beef and cook until browned. Add browned meat to a slow cooker.
2. In the same skillet used to cook the ground meat, heat the onion, bell

pepper, zucchini, squash, mushrooms, and garlic until just softened, or about 3-4 minutes. Add to the slow cooker along with the meat.
3. Add tomato paste, chopped tomatoes, wine, and spices, and stir properly.
4. Cover and cook on a low heat for 6-7 hours.

Nutritional Information (per serving): Calories 291.1, total fat 6.4g, sodium 91.3mg, total carbs 28g, dietary fiber 7.2g, protein 21.4g.

Slow Cooker Bolognese Sauce

This sauce has a distinct, rich, meaty flavor.

Serves: 8

Ingredients: 4 slices bacon (slice into small pieces), 1 tablespoon olive oil, 1 medium yellow onion (diced), 1 carrot (chopped fine), 2 celery stalks (chopped fine), 1 pound ground beef (lean), ½ cup tomato paste (no salt added), ½ cup milk (reduced fat), 1½ cups beef stock (low sodium), ½ cup red wine, 1 teaspoon dried basil, 1 teaspoon dried oregano, freshly ground black pepper (to taste).

Cooking Instructions:

1. Sauté bacon in a large frying pan for 5 minutes over a medium heat. Add the olive oil, onion, carrots, and celery, and cook for another 5-6 minutes. Add the ground beef to the pan and cook until browned, stirring occasionally, for about 4-5 minutes.
2. Add the tomato paste, milk, beef stock, and red wine to a slow cooker. Stir properly to dissolve the tomato paste. Add the meat mixture to the slow cooker. Season with salt and pepper.

3. Cover and cook on a low heat for 6 hours.

Nutritional Information (per serving): Calories 175, total fat 9g, sodium 157mg, total carbs 7g, protein 15g.

Mexican Beef Stew

This hearty stew is a flavorful twist on the traditional beef stew.

Serves: 6

Ingredients: 1 pound beef stew meat, slice into 1-inch cubes, 2 tablespoons all-purpose flour, 1 tablespoon olive oil, 1 15-ounce can black beans (no salt-added, rinsed and drained), 2 medium carrots (sliced), 1 medium onion (chopped), 2 cloves garlic (minced), 1 14.5-ounce can diced tomatoes (no salt added), 1 14.5-ounce can low-sodium beef broth, 2 teaspoon chili powder, 1 teaspoon ground cumin, ½ teaspoon freshly ground black pepper, ½ teaspoon crushed red pepper, 1 cup frozen corn kernels, 1 avocado, (peeled, pitted, and cubed–optional).

Cooking Instructions:

1. Place the beef cubes in a bowl, sprinkle with flour. Stir to coat beef with flour.
2. Heat the olive oil in a skillet over a medium-high heat. Add the beef cubes and brown beef on all sides, for 5 minutes.

3. Add the beef, beans, carrots, onion, garlic, diced tomatoes, beef broth, and spices to a slow cooker. Stir to combine.
4. Cover and cook on low for 7 hours or until the beef is tender.
5. Add the corn kernels and stir gently. Cover and cook for another 15 minutes.
6. Serve topped with avocado cubes.

Nutritional Information (per serving): Calories 272, total fat 9g, sodium 456mg, total carbs 27g, dietary fiber 7.8g, protein 22g.

Moroccan Beef Tagine

Cooking this dish in the slow cooker allows the flavors to deepen and develop.

Serves: 4 to 6

Ingredients: For the spice rub: 1 tablespoon cumin, 1 tablespoon cinnamon, 1 tablespoon ginger, 1 tablespoon paprika, 1 teaspoon nutmeg, 1 teaspoon turmeric, ½ teaspoon sea salt, 1 teaspoon freshly ground black pepper. For the stew: 1½ pounds stew beef, 2 tablespoons olive oil, 1 medium onion (chopped), 1 bunch fresh coriander, 1 14-ounce can chopped tomatoes, 3 cups vegetable or beef stock (low-sodium), 1 small zucchini (chopped), 1 large carrot (sliced thin), 1 red bell pepper (sliced thin), 3-4 prunes (chopped), freshly ground black pepper (to taste).

Cooking Instructions:

1. In a small bowl mix together all of the ingredients for the spice rub.
2. Place the beef in a large zip lock bag. Add the spice mixture and shake to thoroughly coat the meat. Put in a

refrigerator for a couple of hours or overnight.
3. Heat the olive oil in a large skillet over a medium heat. Add the beef and brown on all sides, for about 5 minutes.
4. Add the meat to a slow cooker. Add all the remaining ingredients. Stir to combine.
5. Cover and cook on a high heat for 5-6 hours, or a low heat for 7-8 hours.

Nutritional Information (per serving): Calories 338, total fat 17g, sodium 329mg, total carbs 18g, protein 26g.

Lamb Tagine with Pears

Tagines are slow-cooked meats, vegetables, and fruits that are easily adapted to a slow cooker.

Serves: 5

Ingredients: 1 tablespoon olive oil, 2 medium onions (sliced), 2 pounds lamb meat (slice into 1 to 2 inch cubes), 2 teaspoons cumin, 2 teaspoons coriander, 1 teaspoon ginger, 1 teaspoon cinnamon, 1 teaspoon freshly ground black pepper (to taste), 1½ cups chicken broth (low-sodium), 1 bay leaf, 1 tablespoon lemon juice, 4 pears (peeled and cored – slice into 1 inch cubes), ½ cup golden raisins, ½ cup slivered almonds (blanched).

Cooking Instructions:

1. Heat the olive oil in a large skillet over a medium heat, add the onions and sauté for 2-3 minutes. Add in the lamb meat and continue to cook, stirring, until the lamb is browned on all sides. Add the lamb and onions to a slow cooker.
2. Season with cumin, coriander, ginger, cinnamon, and black pepper. Pour in chicken broth, and add in a bay leaf and

lemon juice. Cover and cook on a low heast for 6-7 hours, or a high heat for 4-5 hours, or until the meat is tender.
3. Add in the pears, raisins, and almonds, cover and cook on low for another 15 minutes, or until the pears are soft.
4. Serve over couscous.

Nutritional Information (per serving): Calories 394, total fat 14.5g, sodium 246mg, total carbs 42g, dietary fiber 7.5g, protein 26.5g.

Slow-Cooker Beef Stew Provencal

Serves: 10

Ingredients: Bouquet garni, cheesecloth, 1 bay leaf, 1 stalk celery (chopped), 3 sprigs fresh parsley, 3 sprigs fresh thyme stew, 2 tablespoons extra-virgin olive oil (divided), 3 pounds beef chuck (or other stew meat, slice into 1-inch pieces), 3 teaspoons kosher salt (divided), ½ teaspoon freshly ground pepper (divided), 3 medium yellow onions (chopped), 4 cloves garlic (minced), 3-4 large carrots (sliced into 1-inch rounds), 3 tablespoons tomato paste (no salt added), 1 pound mushrooms (sliced), 1 quart beef stock (low-sodium), ¼ cup red wine.

Cooking Instructions:

1. To assemble the bouquet garni, slice a square of cheesecloth, then place the bay leaf, celery, parsley, and thyme in the center. Tie with kitchen twine.
2. To prepare the stew heat 1 tablespoon olive oil in a large heavy-duty pan. Add the beef cubes and cook until browned on all sides. Transfer to a slow cooker, season with 1 teaspoon salt and black pepper.

3. Add another tablespoon of oil to pan and add onions, garlic, and carrots. Cook, stirring occasionally until they begin to soften, for about 4-5 minutes. Season with the remaining salt and pepper. Add to the slow cooker with beef.
4. Add tomato paste, mushrooms, beef stock, red wine, and bouquet garni to the slow cooker. Stir to combine.
5. Cover and cook on a low setting for 8-9 hours or a high setting for 5-6 hours.

Nutritional Information (per serving): Calories 351, sodium 380mg, protein 26g, carbs 14g, dietary fiber 5g, fat 15g.

Slow-Cooked Beef Roast

Serves: 8

Ingredients: 1 tablespoon olive oil, 1 chuck beef roast (3 pounds), ½ teaspoon salt, 1 teaspoon black pepper, 2 cups low-sodium beef broth, 6 large carrots (sliced), 3 medium onions (diced), 2 cups mushrooms (sliced), 3 cloves garlic (minced), 3 stalks celery (diced), 2 tablespoons tomato paste, 1 tablespoon Worcestershire sauce, 2 sprigs fresh thyme, 2 tablespoons all-purpose flour.

Cooking Instructions:

1. Heat the oil in a large skillet over a medium-high heat. Sprinkle the roast with salt and pepper. Place the roast in a pan and brown on all sides, for about 5 minutes. Put the roast in a slow cooker.
2. Add remaining ingredients except for the flour. Stir, cover, and cook on low for 7-8 hours or high for 3-4 hours, until the roast is cooked through.
3. Remove a ¼ cup of broth from the slow cooker and place in small bowl. Add flow and mix until the flour is dissolved. Add back into slow cooker and stir. Remove and discard the thyme sprigs.

4. Slice roast and top with vegetables and sauce.

Nutritional Information (per serving): Calories 284, sodium 424mg, protein 31g, carbohydrates 17g, dietary fiber 1.5g, fat 9g.

Beef Stew with Butternut Squash

This aromatic stew with just a hint of sweetness is perfect for a crisp autumn day.

Serves: 4

Ingredients: 3 tablespoons olive oil, 1 medium yellow onion (diced), 3 cloves garlic (minced), 2 pounds stew beef (slice into cubes), 1 16-ounces can diced tomatoes (no salt added), 1 large butternut squash (trimmed and sliced into bite-size cubes), 4 cups beef broth (low-sodium), 1 tablespoon rosemary, 1 tablespoon thyme, freshly ground black pepper (to taste).

Cooking Instructions:

1. Heat the olive oil in a large pot over a medium heat. Add the onions and garlic and sauté for 2-3 minutes. Add the beef cubes and cook until the beef is browned, for about 5 minutes.
2. Transfer to a slow cooker. Add the diced tomatoes, butternut squash, beef broth, rosemary, and thyme. Set cooker to a low setting and cook for 8 hours. Add the salt and freshly ground black pepper to taste.

Nutritional Information (per serving): Calories 580, sodium 292mg, protein 51g, carbohydrates 8g, fat 36g.

Irish Stew

This is a hearty stew.

Serves: 6-8

Ingredients: 2 pounds lamb roast, slice into 1-inch pieces, 1 pound small red potatoes (slice into bite-size pieces), 1 medium onion (sliced), 2 large carrots (sliced), 1 large parsnip (sliced), 3 stalks celery (chopped), 3 cups chicken broth (low sodium), 2 teaspoon fresh thyme (chopped), ½ teaspoon sea salt, 1 teaspoon pepper.

Cooking Instructions:

1. Combine all ingredients in a slow cooker. Stir to combine.
2. Cover and cook on low for 8 hours.

Nutritional Information (per serving): Calories 269, sodium 257mg, protein 39g, carbohydrates 20g, fat 7g.

Cider Pork Roast

This is a very tender and full-flavored pork roast.

Serves: 8

Ingredients: 1 teaspoon ground ginger, ¼ teaspoon salt, ½ teaspoon freshly ground black pepper, 3 tablespoons all-purpose flour, 1 pork loin roast (3 pounds), 1 tablespoon olive oil, 1 medium yellow onion (chopped), 1 apple (peeled, cored, and chopped), 3 cloves (garlic, minced), 2 stalks celery (chopped), 4 carrots (sliced), 2 cups apple cider, 1½ cups water.

Cooking Instructions:

1. Combine the ginger, salt, pepper, and flour in a bowl. Sprinkle the flour mixture over roast, covering all sides.
2. In a large skillet, heat the oil over a medium-high heat. Add the roast and brown on all sides, for about 5 minutes.
3. Place the roast in a slow cooker. Add all the remaining ingredients. Cover and cook on a low heat for 6-7 hours, or on a high heat for 3-4 hours, or until the pork is cooked through.

Nutritional Information (per serving): Calories 235, sodium 125mg, protein 21g, carbohydrates 20g, dietary fiber 2g, fat 8g.

Vegetable Dishes

Baked Potatoes with Broccoli and Mushrooms

You may not think about baking potatoes in a slow cooker but it is an easy way to make them, and they usually come out moist and delicious. These veggie-topped potatoes make a meal in themselves.

Serves: 4

Ingredients: 4 medium baking potatoes (washed), 2 tablespoons olive oil (divided), ½ pound mushrooms (sliced), 1 bunch broccoli (slice into small florets), ⅓ cup broth (vegetable, chicken, or beef, hot, low-sodium), freshly ground black pepper (to taste), ⅔ cup plain yogurt (low-fat).

Cooking Instructions:

1. Make sure the potatoes are completely dry. Rub the potatoes with 1 tablespoon of olive oil. Wrap each potato in aluminum foil. Place in a slow cooker, cover, and cook on a low setting for 7-8 hours or a high setting for 4-5 hours, or until the potatoes are tender.

2. Heat the remaining tablespoon of olive oil in a large skillet over a medium heat. Add the mushrooms and broccoli and sauté until the broccoli is tender, but not soft, for about 10 minutes.
3. Unwrap each potato from the foil. Make a slice in the center of potatoes and scoop out the potato into a bowl. Add the broth, pepper, and yogurt. Mix to combine. Divide mixture and stuff back into potato skins. Top with the broccoli and mushrooms.

Nutritional Information (per serving): Calories 330, total fat 7g, sodium 360mg, total carbs 57g, dietary fiber 8g, protein 14g.

Sweet Potato Coconut Curry

This is a mild curry that makes a delicious side to fish or chicken.

Serves: 4

Ingredients: 1 tablespoon olive oil, 1 small yellow onion (diced), 3 clove garlic (minced), 1 teaspoon cumin powder, ½ teaspoon turmeric, ½ teaspoon cardamom, ½ teaspoon cinnamon, ½ teaspoon ground ginger, 1 14.5-ounce can diced tomatoes (no salt added), 4 medium sweet potatoes (peeled and sliced into bite-size cubes), 1 14-ounce can coconut milk, freshly ground black pepper (to taste), flat leaf parsley for garnish.

Cooking Instructions:

1. Add all ingredients to a slow cooker. Mix to combine. Cover and cook on a low setting for 4-5 hours until the sweet potatoes are tender.
2. Serve hot, topped with fresh parsley for garnish.

Nutritional Information (per serving): Calories 174, total fat 10g, sodium 36mg, total carbs 20g, protein 4g.

Mediterranean Vegetable Stew

This is a really easy stew that makes a nice, light vegetarian meal. Serve over brown rice or orzo.

Serves: 10

Ingredients: 1 butternut squash (peeled and cubed), 1 eggplant (cubed), 1 large zucchini (cubed), 1 medium yellow onion (chopped), 1 tomato (diced) 1 carrot (sliced thin), 2 cloves garlic (minced), 1 cup tomato sauce (low-sodium–homemade or store bought), ½ cup vegetable broth (low-sodium), ½ teaspoon ground cumin, ½ teaspoon turmeric, ½ teaspoon crushed red pepper, ¼ teaspoon cinnamon, ¼ teaspoon paprika.

Cooking Instructions:

1. Combine all ingredients in slow cooker. Stir, cover, and cook on a low heat for 7-8 hours, or a high heat for 4-5 hours, or until the vegetables are tender.

Nutritional Information (per serving): Calories 122, total fat 0.5g, sodium 157mg, total carbohydrates 30g, dietary fiber 7.8g, protein 3.4g.

Slow Cooker Baked Beans

These beans may take a while, but have a taste that is so much more than canned baked beans.

Serves: 8

Ingredients: 1 pound dry great Northern beans, 8 cups water, 4 ounces salt pork (diced), 1 medium yellow onion (chopped), ½ cup molasses, ⅓ cup brown sugar (packed), 1 teaspoon dry mustard, 2 tablespoons cider vinegar, ½ teaspoon freshly ground black pepper.

Cooking Instructions:

1. In a large saucepan, bring the beans and water to the boil. Cook for 2 hours. Place in a pan with beans and water, covered, and leave in the refrigerator overnight.
2. The next day, pour beans and 1½ cups of their liquid into a slow cooker. Add in the salt pork, molasses, brown sugar, dry mustard, and black pepper. Cover and cook on low for 12-14 hours.

Nutritional information (per serving): Calories 365, total fat 12g, sodium 215mg, total carbs 54g, dietary fiber 1.7g, protein 12g.

Moroccan Root Vegetable Tagine

Subtly spiced, this vegetarian dish makes a nice meal served with couscous.

Serves: 8

Ingredients: 1 pound parsnips (peeled and cubed), 1 pound sweet potatoes (peeled and cubed), 2 medium yellow onions (chopped), 1 pound carrots (chopped), 12 dried apricots (chopped), 8 prunes (pitted and chopped), 2 teaspoon turmeric, 2 teaspoon cumin, 1 teaspoon ground ginger, 1 teaspoon cinnamon, ½ teaspoon cayenne pepper, 1 tablespoons dried parsley, 1 tablespoon cilantro, 3 cups vegetable broth (low-sodium).

Cooking Instructions:

1. Place vegetables in a slow cooker. Season with spices and stir to coat. Pour in the vegetable broth.
2. Cover and cook for 5-6 hours on a low heat or 3-4 hours on high, or until vegetables are tender.
3. Serve with couscous.

Nutritional Information (per serving): Calories 171, total fat 0.7g, sodium 188mg, total carbs 38g, dietary fiber 8.7g, protein 3.4g.

Vegetarian Vegetable Stew

This is perfect as a side dish or a light meal.

Serves: 6

Ingredients: 4 large carrots (sliced), 2 medium turnips (peeled and cubes), 1 large onion (sliced thin), 3 garlic cloves (minced), 1 zucchini (sliced), 2 yellow squash (sliced), 2 cups vegetable broth (low-sodium), ½ teaspoon red pepper flakes, 1 teaspoon thyme freshly ground black pepper (to taste).

Cooking Instructions:

1. Combine all ingredients in a slow cooker.
2. Cover, and cook on a low heat for 5-6 hours or on a high heat for 3-4 hours.

Nutritional Information (per serving): Calories 55, total fat 0g, sodium 112mg, total carbs 13g, protein 2g.

WHAT TO EAT, WHEN AND IN WHAT QUANTITIES?

The DASH diet is based on 2,000 calories a day, with the following nutritional profile:

- Total fat: 27% of calories.
- Saturated fat: 6% of calories.
- Protein: 18% of calories.
- Carbohydrate: 55% of calories.
- Cholesterol: 150mg.
- Sodium: 2,300mg.
- Potassium: 4,700mg.
- Calcium: 1,250mg.
- Magnesium: 500mg.
- Fiber: 30g.

These percentages translate into more practical guidelines using food group servings.

Grains and grain products: Seven to eight servings per day. One serving is equivalent to one slice of bread, half a cup of dry cereal, or cooked rice or pasta. These foods provide energy, carbohydrates, and fiber.

Vegetables: Four to five servings per day. One serving size is one cup of leafy vegetables, a half-cup of cooked vegetables, or a half-cup of vegetable juice. Fruits and vegetables provide potassium, magnesium, and fiber. Consuming the full number of vegetable servings is a key component of the diet.

Fruits: Four to five servings per day. One serving is one medium fruit, a half-cup of fruit juice, or one-quarter cup of dried fruit.

Low-fat dairy foods: Two to three servings per day. One serving is equivalent to one cup of milk or yogurt, or one ounce (30g) cheese. Dairy provides rich sources of protein and calcium.

Meat, fish, poultry: Two or fewer servings per day. One serving is 2.5 ounces (75g). The emphasis is on lean meats and skinless poultry. These provide protein and magnesium.

Nuts, seeds, and beans: Four to five servings per week. Portion sizes are half a cup of cooked beans and two tablespoons of seeds. These are good vegetable sources of protein, as well as magnesium and potassium.

Fats and oils: Two to three servings per day. One serving is one teaspoon of oil or soft margarine. Fat choices should be heart healthy unsaturated sources (canola, corn, olive, or sunflower). Saturated and trans fat consumption should be decreased.

Sweets: Five servings per week. A serving is one tablespoon of pure fruit jam, syrup, honey, and sugar. The plan still allows for treats, but the healthier the better.

An example breakfast menu is: cornflakes (one cup) with 1 teaspoon sugar, skim milk (one cup), orange juice (½ cup), a banana, and a slice of whole wheat bread with one tablespoon jam. Suggested snacks during the day include dried apricots (¼ cup), low-fat yogurt (one cup), and mixed nuts (1.5 oz. or 40 g).

These guidelines are available in the National Institutes of Health (NIH) updated booklet, "Your Guide to Losing weight with DASH," which also provides background information, weekly menus, and recipes.

Precautions

Adding high-fiber foods to the diet should be done gradually to avoid side effects such as gas, bloating, and diarrhea. It is important to increase fluid at the same time, as fiber draws water into the bowel. High fiber intake with inadequate fluid can cause hard stools and constipation.

Increasing fruits and vegetables increases the potassium content of the diet. For healthy people with normal kidney function, a higher potassium intake from foods does not pose a risk, as excess potassium is excreted in the urine. However, individuals whose urinary potassium excretion is impaired, such as those with end-stage renal disease, severe heart failure, or adrenal insufficiency, may be at risk of hyperkalemia (high levels of potassium in the blood). Hyperkalemia may cause cardiac arrhythmias (irregular heartbeat), which could be potentially serious. Some common drugs can also decrease potassium excretion. Individuals at risk should consult a doctor before starting the DASH diet, as higher potassium intake in the form of fruit and vegetables may not be suitable. Care should also be taken with potassium-containing salt substitutes.

Risks

Currently, there are no known risks associated with the DASH diet. However, the long-term effects of the diet on morbidity and mortality are still unknown.

Since the original research, scientists also have found that they could apply the DASH diet plan for weight loss. When people follow the DASH diet in addition to increasing exercise, they lose weight and improve metabolic measures such as insulin sensitivity. However, in comparison to low-carbohydrate diets, the DASH diet alone was not as effective a strategy for weight loss. When the DASH diet is followed along with exercise and caloric reduction, people improved their blood pressure even more; lowering it by 16 mmHg systolic and 9mmHg diastolic. In addition to this, they lost some weight. As people adopt the DASH diet and lower their blood pressure, they may have a reduced need for medication. Discuss the diet-based changes you are making with your health-care professional, and if your blood pressure is at or below goal (less than 140/80), you can discuss reducing your medication and maintaining your blood pressure with diet alone.

What is the recommended daily allowance of sodium?

The National Institutes of Health's 2015-2020 Dietary Guidelines for Americans recommend consuming less than 2,300mg of salt each day as part of a healthy diet.

How does the DASH diet lower blood pressure and promote weight loss?

The DASH diet is rich in potassium, magnesium, calcium, and fiber, and also has a low content of sodium (salt) and saturated fats. Adding more of these nutrients improves the electrolyte balance in the body, allowing it to excrete the excess fluid that contributes to high blood pressure. These nutrients also promote relaxation of the blood vessels, reducing the blood pressure. These nutrients are often deficient in overweight and obese people, so the DASH diet can help correct those deficiencies and help people feel better. With the diet alone, some people may lose weight with the DASH diet, but most will need to add exercise or further reduce carbohydrates to see big weight losses. The good news for people with diabetes, prediabetes, or insulin resistance is that the DASH diet does improve insulin sensitivity.

- The DASH diet guidelines from the original research study specified two levels of sodium reduction.
- The DASH diet phase 1 limited sodium to 2300mg, or about 1 teaspoon per day.
- The DASH diet phase 2 further reduced sodium to 1500mg.

To reach the goal of phase 2, the person should avoid all table salt and avoid adding any salt to cooking. We tend to get more than the recommended amount of sodium when we eat packaged or processed foods, or when eating or dining out. Salt is the major source of sodium in the diet, and we can usually refer to the two words interchangeably unless we are discussing specific biochemical processes.

DASH Diet and Weight Loss: How to Cut Calories From Your Day

What foods are allowed in the DASH diet eating plan?

People often ask what foods are on the DASH diet eating plan. The good news is that it includes a wide variety of foods, and many options. The DASH diet is simple. Eat more fruit, and especially vegetables, and eat fewer foods high in salt (sodium). For example:

- Eat a salad with protein for lunch instead of a burger and fries.
- Choose low-fat dairy products such as Greek yogurt instead of fruity, sweetened yogurt.
- Choose snacks such as fruit, raw veggie sticks, bean-based spreads like hummus or black bean dip, and raw unsalted nuts.
- Whole grains are encouraged, such as brown rice or quinoa along with lean proteins such as chicken, lean pork, and fish.

What foods and drinks should be avoided while following a DASH diet?

Foods and drinks to avoid when following the DASH diet include highsugar, high-fat snacks, and foods high in salt such as:

- Candy
- Cookies
- Chips

- Salted nuts
- Sodas
- Sugary beverages
- Pastries
- Snacks
- Meat dishes
- Prepackaged pasta and rice dishes (excluding macaroni and cheese because it is a separate category)
- Pizza
- Soups
- Salad dressings
- Cheese
- Cold cuts and cured meats
- Breads and rolls
- Sandwiches
- Sauces and gravies

Using a salt substitute made with potassium not only works as a substitute in cooking and on the table, but the additional potassium can help lower blood pressure. People who are on blood pressure medications that increase potassium should ask their doctors to help them monitor the blood level of potassium (K) while they are making changes.

What about red meat and heart disease?

While not specifically recommended, grass-fed beef and buffalo would fit within these parameters. Grass-fed beef has a very different composition than conventional grain-fed beef. Grass-fed beef is high in omega-3s and is more similar to fish, nutritionally. Grain-fed red meat is high in omega 6s and saturated fat, both of which are promote inflammation and contribute to heart disease, high blood pressure, and obesity. Red meat that is not grass-fed is not permitted.

What is a sample DASH diet sample menu?

A typical 1600 calorie DASH diet menu plan would include the following:

- 2 cups of vegetables.
- 2 servings of fruit.
- 2 servings of low-fat/fat-free dairy products.
- 6 oz whole grains (1 slice multi-grain bread plus 1 small serving of brown rice).
- 5 oz lean meat, poultry or fish (the size of 1½ playing cards).
- 2 teaspoons healthy oils, such as olive oil.
- 1 oz nuts and seeds.

Rare, mini servings of sweets, salty foods, and alcohol (once a week).

A typical daily DASH diet sample menu might look like this:

Breakfast: Steel cut oatmeal with chopped pecans, half a chopped apple and cinnamon, black coffee.

Morning snack: Other half of the apple with 1 teaspoon peanut butter, large glass of water.

Lunch: Spring greens salad with mixed vegetables, grilled chicken breast and vinaigrette dressing on the side. Dip your fork in the dressing to get flavor with every bite without saturating the salad with salt and fat. Drink unsweetened iced tea or water.

Afternoon snack: Unsweetened fruity iced tea or carrot sticks with hummus.

Dinner: Spiralizer-made zucchini pasta with marinara made with ground turkey and Italian spices, sparkling mineral water.

Dessert: Strawberries, 1 tablespoon vanilla yogurt, dusting of cocoa powder.

What are some DASH diet recipes?
Breakfast

Whole grain toast, avocado, smoked salmon.

Night before muesli - in a glass refrigerator container combine equal parts quick oats, unsweetened coconut flakes, raw sunflower seeds, and frozen blueberries. Mix and cover with unsweetened almond/oat/coconut milk or low-fat dairy milk if you aren't lactose intolerant.

Lunch

Make it easy. Make your lunch a salad plus protein and enjoy the millions of variations on the theme.

From home: leftover roasted veggies and grilled chicken on a bed of butter lettuce, with extra-virgin olive oil and quality balsamic vinegar and chopped walnuts drizzled on top.

If you are out: A mixed greens salad, hold the cheese, add chicken, a hard-boiled egg, or grass-fed steak. Put the dressing on the side, and dip your fork in to get flavor with each bite without overdoing it.

Dinner

Keep it simple. Focus on a healthy full-flavored vegetable recipe, complement it with protein, and add a side of whole grains.

Brown rice pilaf made with pine nuts, celery, onion, and herbs de Provence.

Grilled wild salmon with cracked pepper.

Steamed broccolini with a small pat of butter or olive oil drizzle.

Snacks

Fresh fruit and nuts and small servings of low-fat dairy are the mainstays of the DASH diet snacks.

How can I make the DASH diet tastier?

While the DASH diet includes solid nutrition recommendations, it can be hard for someone new to these recommendations to make food palatable. We are used to sugar and salt as the major "flavors" of our meals. To make the healthy foods in the DASH diet more appealing, be generous with herbs and spices. There are a number of salt-free spice blends that can be used for many recipes. Some options include herbs de Provence blends, Italian herb blend, Indian curry blend, and Baja fish taco blend (check that they are salt-free or you are derailing your good efforts).

These spice blends can be sprinkled on proteins while grilling, turned into a salad dressing with extra-virgin olive oil and white wine vinegar, or sprinkled on a sandwich to reduce the mayonnaise or cheese we typically add for flavor.

What heart-healthy lifestyle interventions are part of the DASH diet?

While the original DASH diet research didn't include other lifestyle changes, it makes sense to include them, and the combination has since been researched and shown to be effective.

Physical activity, weight loss and high blood pressure

It is important to be physically active every day, such as taking a walk after dinner. The more activity and exercise a person does, the more benefits the body receives. As we exercise, the muscles demand oxygen, and nitric oxide is released to relax the blood vessels to allow more blood and oxygen in. Over time, this becomes a permanent effect, lowering the blood pressure even when you are not physically active. For blood pressure and weight loss, physical activity should include regular walking, dancing, swimming, cycling, or other cardiovascular (aerobic) activity, but it also should include some strength training. Building more muscle through weight or strength training has the best effect on weight loss and increasing metabolism.

Weight management and high blood pressure

Losing weight is difficult for most people, but it ultimately improves more than just your blood pressure. With weight loss, most cardiovascular (heart) risk factors improve, your risk for cancers, diabetes, dementia, and many other chronic diseases lessen. Social support is very important to be successful in weight loss. Make a commitment with several friends or join a program that helps keep you accountable and provides support. If you are struggling to lose weight despite eating a DASH diet and being physically active, there might be problems with your metabolism or other underlying factors. Discuss the situation with your health care professional to see if other conditions may be impacting your metabolism.

Alcohol use and high blood pressure

Alcohol increases blood pressure and should be consumed in moderation in the DASH diet plan. The recommendations for alcohol are to limit it to one drink per day for women, and two per day for men.

Stress management and high blood pressure

Stress can raise blood pressure even if you are following a healthy DASH diet plan. Many times, the things that cause stress are outside of our control and we feel we cannot change it (stress at work, family situations, or health worries). What we can change is how we let stress impact us. By learning to be more stress resilient, we can reduce the impact of stress, such as high blood pressure and weight gain. Stress management techniques, such as courses in meditation (which can be found online or in person), are a good option. Two types of mediation, transcendental meditation and mindfulness-based stress reduction, have been studied and proven to lower blood pressure as well as increase peace of mind and stress resiliency.

Mind and body exercises such as yoga and Tai Chi also may help decrease stress. Check with your health care professional if one of these is an option for you.

Sleep and high blood pressure

You may not have realized that poor sleep increases blood pressure. For example, people who have sleep apnea have higher blood pressure than those without the condition, and when that is treated (using a device to ease breathing), the blood pressure is reduced.

Smoking and high blood pressure

Smoking raises the blood pressure, as well as contributing to other chronic diseases. It is difficult to quit smoking, so ask for help if you need it. Options to help you quit range from support groups to medications and hypnosis.

HOW TO LOSE WEIGHT IN SEVEN DAYS BY EATING

The overall goal of the DASH Diet is to lower your consumption of sodium, which aids in lowering your blood pressure. Since the diet focuses on eating the right foods with the right portions, it's also effective for short- and long-term weight loss, and even during menopause for women.

Phase 1: Two Weeks to Lose Weight by Eating

To regulate your blood sugar and help curb your cravings, avoid fruit and whole grains, which have a lot of natural sugar, and alcohol, which also contain sugars. With this said, you can still enjoy 2-3 servings of low-fat dairy per day. This would include 1 cup of skim milk or low-fat yogurt. Avoid regular or even fat-free cheese because they are often high in sodium.

By avoiding starchy foods with sugar, you're helping to regulate your blood sugar and diminish cravings. Try leafy greens like lettuce and spinach or cruciferous vegetables like broccoli or cabbage. You can also eat cucumbers, squash, peppers, and tomatoes.

You can also enjoy up to 6 ounces of lean meats, fish, and poultry a day. Aim for 4 to 5 servings of beans or lentils a week.

Opt for protein-rich foods that have healthy fats, like fresh nuts and seeds, or fatty fish like salmon or mackerel. Avocados are loaded with monounsaturated fats as well as the antioxidants lutein, vitamin E and beta-carotene. Toss them in a salad along with vegetable oils, especially olive, canola and nut oils, which you can use as a salad dressing.

Phase 2: Kick It Up a Notch!

After the first 14 days, you will continue to eat the foods from phase 1, but re-introduce some other healthy foods that will help you continue your weight loss. How long does phase 2 last?

It is your life plan and it should last forever, so you can keep your blood pressure low and keep weight off.

Whole Grains: Choose from cereals, breads, and pasta. Aim for 6 to 8 servings a day.

Fruit: Make fruit (fresh or frozen) a part of your daily diet. Aim for 4 to 5 servings a day, and try making low-sugar fruits part of your diet.

Low-Fat Milk or Yogurt: Stick to 2 to 3 servings a day as in Phase 1.

Sugar: You can have 3 to 4 servings of sugary foods each week.

Alcohol: You can have a small glass of red wine occasionally, which represents one fruit serving.

The next page has a week's worth of meals. Phase 1 has 3 sample days, and phase 2 has 4 sample days.

Phase 1: 7 Days to Lose Weight by Eating

Day 1
Breakfast

Hard-boiled egg. (Hint: You can make several hard-boiled eggs, and peel. Store in a zipper bag in the refrigerator. Then you will have them when you need them for super-quick breakfasts. You can also find prepackaged, peeled hard-boiled eggs in some stores).

- 1 or 2 slices Canadian bacon
- 6 ounces tomato juice, low-sodium
- Midmorning Snack
- 1 stick light cheese
- Baby carrots

Lunch

- Quinoa meatless balls
- Cherry tomatoes
- Small side salad: dressed with Italian or oil and vinegar dressing
- Strawberry Jell-O cup, sugar-free

Mid-Afternoon Snack

- 4 ounces lemon light yogurt, fat-free, artificially sweetened.
- 18 cashews (1 ounce by weight, ¼ cup by volume, or small handful).

Before-Dinner Snack (Optional)

Pepper strips. (Hint: To make the strips quickly, cut off the tops and bottoms of some red, yellow, or orange bell peppers. Remove seeds and cut in half. Flatten each half and take a very sharp knife and cut along the surface, removing the membranes. Then cut into 1-inch strips. These are great to dip into guacamole, as a chip substitute).

2 ounces guacamole, which is about ¼ cup.

Dinner

Mediterranean-style chicken kebabs.

1 cup (or more) mixed carrots, broccoli, and cauliflower blend: steamed or microwaved.

Salad: Romaine blend with Italian dressing.

Raspberry Jell-O cup, sugar-free.

Day 2
Breakfast

Mini-egg beaters southwestern style omelet. Spray microwave-safe dish or cup with cooking spray. Add ¼-½ cup egg beaters southwestern style. Microwave on high for 1 minute. Stir, and cook an additional 15 seconds.

4-6 ounces tomato juice, low-sodium.

Mid-Morning Snack

1 light cheese wedge

6 grape tomatoes

Lunch

2-3 Turkey-Swiss roll-ups. Cheese on the outside, as the wrap. Deli turkey slices for the meat. Add whatever condiments you like, such as mustard. You could also add lettuce as the outermost layer of the wrap.

½-1 cup coleslaw.

Raw snow peas or sugar snap pea pods (as much as you like).

Orange Jell-O cup, sugar-free.

Mid-Afternoon Snack

1 stick light cheese.

Baby carrots.

Before-dinner snack (optional).

10 peanuts in the shell (20 individual peanuts) (Hint: Shelling nuts slows you down, so you are less likely to overeat them.)

Dinner

Roasted sliced turkey

Sautéed carrots and onions. Sauté 1 medium onion, thinly sliced, in 1 tablespoon olive oil or canola oil. Add about 8 ounces of sliced carrots, and continue to sauté until the carrots are soft. Add 1 thin pat of butter at the end. (Hint: Top the turkey with the sautéed carrots for extra flavor. If you like very soft carrots, microwave first before sautéing.)

Side salad topped with Italian dressing.

Lime Jell-O cup, sugar-free.

Day 3
Breakfast

Scrambled eggs

1-2 slices Canadian bacon

4-6 ounces diet cranberry juice

Mid-Morning Snack

4 ounces raspberry light yogurt, nonfat, artificially sweetened

23 almonds (1 ounce by weight, cup by volume)

Lunch

Cold fried chicken breast, but don't eat the skin or coating (Hint: The chicken doesn't have to be cold. This could be a fast-food lunch but only if you can choose whole chicken parts.) Definitely do not choose chicken tenders, patties, crispy chicken, or nuggets. They have too much breading for the amount of meat. Most fried chicken places have coleslaw as a side. When you get back to your office, you can have the carrots and Jell-O.

Coleslaw

Baby carrots

Lemon Jell-O cup, sugar-free

Mid-Afternoon Snack

1-2 light cheese wedges

6 grape tomatoes

Before-dinner snack (optional)

Pepper strips

Guacamole

Dinner

Turkey burger

1 cup broccoli

Side salad with balsamic dressing

1-2 strawberry Jell-O cups, sugar-free

Day 5
Breakfast

¾ cup Wheaties (1 ounce by weight)

8 ounces skim milk

4-6 ounces strawberries or raspberries

Mid-Morning Snack (Optional)

1-2 light cheese wedges

Grape tomatoes

Lunch

2-3 turkey and Swiss roll-ups

Baby carrots

Small plum

Mid-Afternoon Snack

6 ounces blueberry light yogurt

10 cashews

Before-Dinner Snack (Optional)

10 peanuts in the shell (20 individual peanuts)

Dinner

Pan-seared tilapia. Heat 1 tablespoon olive oil in a skillet over a medium-high heat. Cook for about 4 minutes per side, or until the fish flakes easily with a fork. Before finishing, place about 1 pat of butter or margarine in the pan, and allow the melted butter to coat all the pieces. (To serve four, choose four 4-ounce tilapia filets.)

Mango-melon salsa

Fresh asparagus

Strawberry Jello-O cup, sugar-free

Day 6
Breakfast

Hot chocolate. To 8 ounces skim milk, add 1 heaping teaspoon unsweetened cocoa and 2 packets Splenda or Truvia.

1-2 hard-boiled eggs

6-8 ounces light cranberry juice. (Hint: Light cranberry juice has more calories than the diet version, but you may prefer it.)

4-6 ounces strawberries

Mid-Morning Snack (Optional)

6 ounces key lime light yogurt, nonfat, artificially sweetened.

10 ounces almonds

Lunch

Turkey and Swiss sandwich. Put 2-4 ounces turkey and a slice of reduced-fat Swiss cheese on two pieces light whole-wheat bread; add lettuce, tomato, and any other veggies or condiments that you choose.

Pepper strips

Coleslaw or side salad

Raspberry Jell-O cup, artificially sweetened.

Mid-Afternoon Snack

1 clementine orange

1-2 light cheese wedges

Before-dinner Snack (optional)

Pepper strips

¼-½ cup hummus

Dinner

Vegetable stir-fry with quinoa

Side salad, with Italian, oil and vinegar, or vinaigrette dressing

Fudge bar

Day 7
Breakfast

½ cup oatmeal, cooked, topped with cinnamon, Splenda Brown Sugar Blend, or Truvia, and 1 tablespoon chopped almonds (optional).

½ banana, medium or large.

4-6 ounces tomato juice, low-sodium.

Latte: 8 ounces skim milk, 2 ounces espresso.

Mid-Morning Snack (Optional)

1 stick light cheese

Baby carrots

Lunch

Three-bean kale sautéed with brown rice

Sliced bell peppers

Orange Jello-O cup, artificially sweetened

Mid-Afternoon Snack

4-6 ounces strawberries

10 cashews

Before-Dinner Snack (Optional)

10 peanuts in the shell (20 individual peanuts)

Dinner

White bean and cabbage soup

Green beans

Sliced tomatoes

Side salad, with Italian dressing

4-6 ounces raspberries on ½-1 cup frozen yogurt, nonfat, artificially sweetened.

EMPTY THE PANTRY AND CHANGE EATING HABITS

Motivation to Change: Life is a beautiful and wondrous experience, the extra sweetenings are also enjoyable. If there are people who care about you, such as children, a spouse, family, friends, or even a pet, think about how their lives would be affected if you were not there. Think of what it would be like for them to see you suffer with illness and even die.

When you compare the look in your child's eyes when she kisses you goodnight, to the taste of a chocolate glazed doughnut or a hamburger, it is obvious which one is superior, and which one is more important.

You deserve to be there for the ones who love you, and you also deserve to be there for yourself. There are so many things in life to see, learn and do. There are places to go, and people to meet. The world is waiting for you and your gifts. Why leave it before your time?

Cleaning Out the Kitchen: After about a week of transitioning into the higher fiber diet, you should be ready to fully commit to the DASH diet plan. Now it is time to rid your kitchen of all the high-fat, high-sodium, low-nutrient foods.

This is an essential step for several reasons. The obvious reason is that when you clean the kitchen out of all unhealthy foods, those foods will no longer be available for you to eat. The less obvious reason is that when you do this ritual, it is a signal to your subconscious that you are serious about improving your health.

First look in the refrigerator. Take out all the full-fat dairy products. This includes milk, yogurt, cheese, cottage cheese, and similar. Next, you are going to get rid of any high-fat red meats. Meats you can leave are chicken and fish, lean beef and pork. Any processed cheeses must go. In fact, most processed foods must go. Get rid of high-sodium condiments such as soy sauce, teriyaki sauce, ketchup, and salad dressings. Check the labels for sodium and fat content. Anything that has 5-6% or more of the daily allowance of sodium per serving should be removed.

What can remain in the refrigerator are fruits and vegetables, low-fat dairy, and lean meats. Anything that does not meet that criteria is to be avoided.

From the freezer, remove any ice cream, TV dinners, and frozen sweets. What can remain are frozen, no-salt-added fruits and vegetables, lean meats, low-sodium veggie-burgers, low-fat frozen yogurt, soy ice cream, or rice ice cream, and similar produce.

Next, go to the pantry. Get rid of any white rice, white bread, refined pastas, chips, crackers, cakes, cookies, and anything that is a refined, simple carbohydrate. Also remove candy and soda. Always remember to check the labels.

You will have to get rid of most canned foods because they usually contain high levels of sodium and fat. Foods such as canned chilies and many types of canned soups commonly have MSG added. Check the labels for MSG and sodium content, and remove anything that has a sodium content of more than 100mg per serving. Be sure to take out anything containing MSG.

The foods that can remain in the pantry are whole-grain foods such as brown or wild rice, whole-grain bread, quinoa, whole-grain pasta, oatmeal, millet, and barley. You can keep canned beans that have no salt added. You can also keep all your dried beans, lentils, and other legumes.

By now the kitchen should be quite different, and it may look completely empty. Try not to think of the wasted money because the amount of money you will save in the long run by protecting your health will be considerable.

Grocery Guide: Shopping for the DASH diet is easy and fun filled, if you follow some simple guidelines.

1. The First Thing You Need to Do Before You Go Shopping is Prepare.

Make a list of the ingredients you will need for your meal plan for the next several days or week. Include all the foods you will need, including snacks and breakfast. A good list of everything you plan to eat for the coming days is the best way to save money, and to stick to your diet plan. Without a list, it is easy to veer away from your plan into tempting, unhealthy foods.

Don't go shopping hungry, and make sure you have eaten before going to the grocery store. The best way to end up with a bunch of unnecessary and unhealthy foods is to go to the store hungry because at these times everything looks appetizing.

2. Remember What the DASH Diet is All About.

The DASH diet is predominantly a diet of fresh, whole foods, so when you go shopping, concentrate on freshness. The less processed foods the better. That means you aim for the organic produce, poultry, seafood, and diary sections. You should concentrate most of your time in the produce department. Fresh foods are full of nutrients, like vitamins and minerals, and are also high in fiber. Those are all the things you need when eating the DASH diet. You should stay away from frozen foods like pizzas, lunch meats, and food in cans.

The fresh food sections are usually around the perimeter of the grocery store.

Read the labels. This can't be emphasized enough. The majority of Americans eat processed foods but have no idea what is in them. Get comfortable with taking an extra minute to read the label and be aware of what you are buying. There is often hidden sodium in many products, so stick to low-sodium, low-fat, low-calorie products.

3. Keep DASH Diet-Friendly Items in the House.

Fruit is one of the best staples to have around the house because it can easily become a substitute for unhealthy sweets. Fruits such as bananas, oranges, apples, grapes and dried/unsweetened fruits are great for snacking and adding to salads.

Vegetables are not always everyone's first choice, but after a while they can become much more appealing. The best approach to take with vegetables is to have a wide variety. The greater the variety, the more flavors you will get to enjoy. Vegetables like tomatoes, carrots, lettuce, mushrooms, broccoli, mixed greens, and spinach are great staples to have around the house for everyday cooking.

Whole grains will become a large part of your diet and can be nicely mixed together with salad vegetables. You need to have a variety of whole grains on hand for different flavors. Some great examples of whole-grain foods are brown and wild rice, whole-grain bread, quinoa, millet, whole-grain cereal, oatmeal and more. Explore the world of whole grains.

Legumes, seeds, and nuts are an important protein source with the DASH diet. Beans such as kidney beans and navy beans are packed with protein. Lentils are an excellent source of iron and make a very hearty soup. Seeds like sunflower seeds are a lower fat alternative to nuts, which are also a great option. Seeds and nuts are excellent to add to raw salad meals. When choosing nuts and seeds, make sure you get unsalted or low-salt varieties.

Lean meats, fish and poultry will round out your protein needs. It is best to stick to poultry and fish. Choose skinless chicken or turkey. Fish is naturally low in fat. Extra lean ground beef is an option, as are round and sirloin beef cuts, in addition to pork tenderloin.

Low-fat dairy products such as low-fat or non-fat milk, low fat kefir, cheese, yogurt and sour cream are permissible on the DASH diet.

Excellent substitutes for table salt are herbs, spices, olive oil, and flavored vinegars, which all add flavor to meals without adding salt.

4. Choose Your Cookware.

Nonstick cookware is a great way to reduce the need for oil or butter when cooking meat or vegetables.

Use a vegetable or rice steamer instead of a pot to reduce the need for butter or oil.

Using a garlic press or spice mill to make it easier to add flavor without the extra salt.

5. Be Aware of Healthy Cooking Practices.

Add plenty of spices, herbs, garlic, ginger, lemon, flavored vinegar, and peppers to add flavor without adding salt.

Rinse your canned foods like canned vegetables, canned tomatoes, and tuna to rinse away the extra salt in the packing liquid.

Many broths include a great deal of sodium. You can make your own vegetable broth by sautéing mushrooms, onions, and other vegetables with water. Or you can purchase no-sodium broths at stores.

Reduce your meat intake. At first this might be difficult, but after a while you may become comfortable with vegetarian meal options and not miss the meat at all. You can also reduce meat in recipes by simply adding a fraction of the meat the recipe calls for.

DASH Diet Food List

Protein: Skinless chicken breast, skinless turkey breast, lean ground turkey, swordfish, haddock, salmon, tuna, crab, lobster, shrimp, top round steak, top sirloin steak, extra lean ground beef, lean ham, egg whites, trout, soy tofu, low-sodium veggie burgers, low-sodium tempeh, unsweetened soy milk, pork tenderloin.

Fruits and Vegetables: Broccoli, asparagus, lettuce, carrots, mixed greens, kale, mushrooms, spinach, tomatoes, peas, cucumber, onions, cauliflowers, green beans, green peppers, potato, Brussels sprouts, artichoke, cabbage, celery, zucchini, sweet potato, yams, squash, pumpkin, corn, strawberries, melon, apple, orange, kiwi, avocado, artichoke, blueberries, raspberries, papaya, green tea.

Whole Grains: Brown rice, wild rice, couscous, kashi, bulgur, whole-wheat pasta, oatmeal, barley, whole-wheat bread, high-fiber cereal, whole-wheat tortilla, whole-wheat pita, millet bread.

Dairy: Low-fat or fat-free yogurt, low-fat or fat-free, milk, low-fat cottage cheese, low-sodium feta.

Legumes, Nuts, and Seeds: Lentils, black beans, soy beans, navy beans, chickpeas, kidney beans, great northern beans, sunflower seeds, pumpkin seeds, peanuts, peanut butter, walnuts, almonds, flax seed.

Oils: Olive oil, grapeseed oil, flaxseed oil, canola oil.

HOW TO PREPARE/ DEFEAT MENOPAUSAL KILOGRAMS WITH THE DASH DIET

The menopause is a season of life is often a very challenging time for women, one filled with hormonal upheaval, mood changes, temperature dysregulation, and undesirable fluctuations in weight. It is very uncomfortable, but does it have to be?

Numerous books and websites have sought to offer solutions to the maladies of menopause, including ideas, such as herbal treatments, essentials oils, stress reduction techniques, exercise plans, and, of course, hormone therapies. All of these can offer help in various ways, and certainly ease the symptoms. The one area that can have the biggest impact, particularly, in not only easing symptoms but also in delaying menopause, is a healthy diet. What you put in your mouth every single day really matters, and it matters not only during the menopause but also in the years before you even go through the "change."

So, which foods are best? The advice is to eat a well-rounded diet, one that is full of fruits, vegetables, legumes and whole grains. This will ensure you are getting adequate amounts of vitamin A, vitamin E, vitamin B, vitamin C, vitamin D, magnesium, calcium and trace minerals, all of which can ease menopausal discomfort and help keep your bones healthy. omega 3 fatty acids can be another beneficial addition.

Here is a quick "eat this, not that" guide to get you going on a hormone-healthy diet plan.

EAT THIS

Vitamin A: Carrots, red peppers, kale, winter squash, sweet potato (these tubers have estrogen-like effects when eaten), watermelon.

B Vitamins: Fruits, vegetables, poultry, fish, eggs, dairy.

Calcium: Dairy products, plant milks, leafy greens, beans, nuts, tofu, broccoli.

Remember that calcium absorption tends to decrease as we age, and be sure to get a wide range of calcium-containing foods in your diet.

Don't forget that in order to get calcium where you want it (in the bones) it needs its cofactors friends for optimal usage. These nutrients include magnesium, vitamin D, boron, and vitamin K.

Vitamin E: Nuts & seeds (almonds, hazelnuts, peanuts, sunflower seeds), spinach, avocado, butternut squash, mango, sweet potato, tomato. Vitamin E is critical as it stimulates the production of estrogen.

Vitamin C: Oranges, strawberries, broccoli, cauliflower, kale, pineapple, parsley, grapefruit, mango.

Vitamin D: Sunlight, fortified foods, sardines, salmon. It is notoriously hard to get adequate amounts of this nutrient from food and sunlight, especially in temperate regions. In rare cases a supplement is highly recommended.

Magnesium: Nuts, whole grains, spinach, pumpkin seeds, figs, avocado, banana, chocolate.

Vitamin K: Dark leafy greens, Brussels sprouts, cabbage, broccoli, prunes, cucumbers, spring onions.

Boron: Beans, berries, sweet potatoes, figs, prunes, plums, avocado, apples, pears, peaches, grapes, nuts. This trace mineral not only helps calcium get into the bones, but research has also shown it can help balance hormone levels and ease menopausal symptoms.

Manganese: Whole grains, beans, hazelnuts, macadamia nuts, oats.

Omega 3 fatty acids: Salmon, mackerel, sardines, mussels, flaxseed, chia seeds, hemp hearts, walnuts.

AVOID THESE

Here are some specific things to avoid for optimal hormonal support. This may come as no surprise,

- Sugar and other refined carbohydrates
- Fast food
- Factory-farmed animal meats
- Caffeine
- Alcohol

Hopefully you have identified some foods you can start including regularly in your diet that you may not already be eating. Usually we can all identify foods we should remove from our normal routine. Also, note that many of the healthy foods are cross-listed, meaning that they have a host of important nutrients in them. Non-processed foods are a powerhouse of nutrition and may just be the extra boost needed to delay or alleviate irritating hormone-related symptoms.

HOW TO LOSE 10 CENTIMETERS OF WAISTLINE IN 21 DAYS

What Causes Waistline Fat for Women in Menopause?

There are a number of factors that can contribute to a person becoming overweight and developing any of the associated conditions that come with obesity. Each of these will be looked at in more depth throughout this book, but to begin with, a couple of causes of waistline fat that many people overlook or fail to consider.

You could have an effective exercise routine and only eat the healthiest foods, but unless you also target some of these root causes, you could find your progress slowing down, or even coming to a complete halt.

Stress

Chronic stress has become an epidemic in our society, and it can potentially cause a number of health problems for the body. In today's world, faster is better, and we attempt to pack increasingly more obligations into our ever-expanding schedules, which puts us all under a lot of pressure.

One meta-analysis involving 300 studies, found that chronic stress could cause damage to your immune system and in addition to this, a study in the journal 'Appetite' found stressed-out women had a significantly higher waist circumference compared to non-stressed women. This is proof that stress can make you fat, particularly around the Waistline.

When you're stressed, your adrenal glands release hormones, like adrenaline and cortisol, that flood your system and raise your heart rate. This will increase your blood pressure, and even your waistline fat storage. This is because deep abdominal fat contains four times the cortisol receptors than fat under the skin, so high levels of cortisol in the blood not only increases fat accumulation in this area, but also has an enlarging effect on the fat cells themselves.

Cortisol also signals for more glucose to be released into the bloodstream, and when this is not used up by the body, it gets stored as fat. Finally, when cortisol is coupled with sugar, your insulin levels increase. This leads to increased inflammation, which worsens the overall feeling. The sugary foods many people might turn to as a 'pick me up' increase cortisol and adrenalin, and this leads to a continuous vicious cycle.

Dealing with Stress

It is best to try and tackle the stress issues you are aware of if you want to start fighting you waistline fat. The best way to start is by making sure you eat properly, as the right diet can do wonders to reduce the impact of stress on your life. When you eat whole, real foods, you restore balance to insulin, cortisol, and other hormones, as well as blood sugar levels. This helps to reduce the damaging impacts of stress.

If you find that you still have the odd stressful day, there are a number of techniques you can use to cope effectively with the problem, and help tackle what could be at the root of your weight issues. Here are some top stress-tackling tips:

1. Address the underlying biological causes of stress. Mercury toxicity, deficiencies in magnesium and vitamin B12, as well as gluten allergies, could all be changing your brain's chemistry and leading to issues with stress. If you suspect a nutrient deficiency or imbalance, speak to a doctor or Naturopath about getting tested.
2. Actively relax. Engage the powerful forces of the mind on the body, by actively doing something relaxing. Whether that means deep breathing or a simple leisurely walk, find active relaxation that works for you and do it regularly. You should be actively doing something to relax.
3. Move your body. Exercise is a powerful, well-studied way to combat stress and heal the mind. Studies suggest exercise works better than, or equal to, Prozac for treating depression.
4. Sleep. Lack of sleep increases stress hormones, in particular cortisol which

promotes weight gain. Ensure you are able to sleep enough as a priority.

Insulin

Numerous hormones contribute to waistline fat, but none proves more powerful than insulin - your fat storage hormone. High levels of insulin tell the body to gain weight around the waistline, and you become more apple-shaped over time. When you become insulin resistant, your body not only generates, but holds onto that Waistline fat.

However, high insulin levels do not simply exist in a vacuum. They influence other hormones like leptin, your satiety hormone. When insulin blocks leptin, your body thinks it is still hungry even after a big meal. This may be a familiar experience after eating a heavy meal like pizza or pasta.

Develop a fatty liver will generate more inflammation, and anything that causes inflammation will worsen insulin resistance. This can also become a negative cycle.

More than any other food, sugar is responsible for hijacking your brain chemistry and metabolism to create insulin resistance and all its repercussions. It may be surprising to know that the average American consumes twenty-two to thirty teaspoons of sugar every day.

By preventing the insulin surges you can arrest waistline fat storage and cravings.

21-Day Activities to Lose 10 Centimeters of Fat Waistline

Day 1

DASH Recipe: As part of your healthy breakfast or lunch, whip up a delicious and sweet flat-waistline smoothie. These are packed with ingredients that fight waistline fat and reduce bloating, such as blueberries, pineapple, kale, and Greek yogurt—all for under 300 calories.

Workout: There are three versions of this treadmill run. If you are new to running, try the walk/run plan later on. If you wish to increase the speed, use the run faster program.

You can get a head start on Day 2 by prepreparing the overnight oats recipe to enjoy the next morning.

Day 2

DASH Recipe: Last night you prepped this whole-grain recipe, so it's time to meet the easiest waistline-improving breakfast of all time: overnight oats. It doesn't get any better than mixing a few ingredients together before bed and grabbing a spoon when you're ready to eat a delicious breakfast.

Workout: Plank is one of the most effective exercises to target your core and upper body. Here's a 20-minute circuit workout combining six different dynamic variations of the basic plank — remember to stretch your back and arms for a couple of minutes after you've completed all those planks.

Day 3

DASH Recipe: After your sweat session, fuel up with a substantial quinoa and kale salad with many different waistline-busting properties. Quinoa is full of protein to help keep you full, while the fiber in kale will also help aid in slow digestion. Moreover, studies have shown that blueberries and almonds may both help diminish waistline fat. At under 400 calories, this colorful and full-flavored salad is hard to beat.

Workouts: If you want to achieve that flat waistline, cardio intervals should be a regular part of your fitness routine. Short, intense bursts have been proven to melt away fat, especially around your midsection. This 30-minute treadmill workout is a favorite of celebs like Sandra Bullock and Kim Kardashian, and once you hop on the machine it'll be easy to see why.

Note: Start your day with this caffeine-free cranberry and apple cider vinegar shot. A favorite of actress Nikki Reed, this detox drink masks the flavor of digestion-friendly, liver-cleansing apple cider vinegar with pure cranberry juice. The result? A boost of energy whenever you need it.

Day 4

DASH Recipe: Don't be put off by the "salad" description; this warm, wilted cabbage and quinoa dish makes a light, comforting dinner that soothes tummy issues. Each ingredient helps digestion, and the fiber in the chickpeas, cabbage, and quinoa will help you debloat. If you'd like, add a dollop of Greek yogurt for a creamy element and a dose of waistline-helping probiotics.

Workouts: Today's ab workout does double-duty in the flat-waistline department: not only does it target your core to help define ab muscles, but it also builds muscles all over your body, which helps rev up your metabolism to burn more calories throughout the day.

Day 5

DASH Recipe: Is it happy hour yet? Our pineapple mojito can be made sans alcohol, but regardless of whether you leave the rum in or out, the cold-pressed juice contains pineapple and mint, which are both known for their detoxing and debloating benefits.

Workout: You've completed four days of intense workouts that have kept your heart rate up and muscles burning. Today it's time to pull back a bit and allow your body the rest it needs to recharge itself for tomorrow's workout. As any trainer will tell you, a rest day is just as important as a workout.

Don't forget, though, that a day of rest doesn't always have to equal inactivity. Opt for some light cardio like a walk around the neighborhood, which will help get the blood flowing to tired muscles. If that doesn't appeal to you, give your body the stretch it needs by flowing through a restorative yoga sequence or just enjoy a relaxing night in.

Day 6

DASH Recipes: Made with a handful of ingredients you probably already have in your kitchen, today's healthy treat is a cinch to whip up. The berries, almonds, and yogurt in this low-calorie dessert help fight waistline fat with every bite.

Workouts: Today's workout is 30 minutes of steady-state cardio followed by some serious ab work. Pick your favorite cardio — running, cycling, swimming, dancing — and keep moving at a steady pace for 30 minutes. Then strengthen your core and tone your abs with this 10-minute ab video.

Day 7

DASH Recipe: Since wheat can cause bloating for many, make our low-carb, DASH-friendly noodles made from zucchini instead. Lightly cooked until tender and flavored with garlic and red pepper flakes, this grain-free pasta alternative is perfectly filling, but won't leave you feeling stuffed.

Workout: If your body could use some fine-tuning, hop on your yoga mat and do today's eight poses designed to detox the body. You have your circulatory, digestive, and lymphatic systems to thank for getting rid of toxins and waste, and these poses stimulate those systems. Pick out the poses your body needs or practice them all, and you'll be on your way to feeling like a new you.

Day 8

DASH Recipe: Give yourself an energizing reboot while also debloating the waistline with a vegan avocado smoothie. Made with fiber-rich avocado to keep things moving along, it's also made with hydrating aloe vera juice and coconut water, as well as toxin-flushing lemon juice to help keep your digestive system feeling happy.

Workout: It's time to step up your fat-blasting running workout with intervals! Get ready to burn some mega calories with a longer 45-minute treadmill workout. Set the incline to one percent to prevent shin splints, and as with all our workouts, feel free to increase or decrease speed, depending on your level of fitness.

Note: Get ready for Day 9: here's another overnight recipe that takes just a few minutes to prep and is a delicious way to start your morning — chia seed pudding.

Day 9

Workout: Doing the basics of Capoeira, a Brazilian dance-like martial art, will work your waistline, legs, arms, and back from every angle. The 30-minute workout is both challenging and fun, and trainer Brett Hoebel provides modifications for every level. Get ready to sweat and burn some serious calories!

DASH Recipe: Chia seeds and coconut milk marry for a Paleo-friendly pudding that works great for breakfast. High in anti-inflammatory omega-3s, this sweet chia pudding is a make-ahead recipe that will save you time, fill you up on fiber, and help you debloat. This flat-waistline breakfast is full of good-for-you ingredients, but the flavor will make it feel like dessert! Top off your jar with fresh pineapple or your favorite Summer berries for even more flat-waistline power.

Day 10

DASH Recipe: For a quick detoxifying meal, this crunchy cabbage and hemp salad does what you need, deliciously. It's chock full of fiber to help regulate bloating and digestion, and it's easy to throw together on a busy weekday.

Workout: If you're short on time today, this 30-minute elliptical workout is just for you. It gets you in and out of the gym fast, while burning a substantial amount of calories to boot. And since intervals blast waistline fat, this is a great midweek workout to do, especially if you're bored of the treadmill or need to fit in a workout at lunch.

Note: Feeling a bit sluggish? Whip up a chia, supergreens, and coconut water superfoods shot, which is full of fiber and is perfect for a morning boost. Celebrity trainer Valerie Waters recommends her clients chug this drink before a morning workout for an extra energy boost.

Day 11

DASH Recipe: Think of our Summer quinoa salad as a bulked-up tabbouleh, since detoxifying parsley lays the base of the greens, while a scoop of quinoa and diced avocado provide over 60 percent of your daily recommended fiber — a must-have nutrient if you're looking to support healthy digestion and your flat-waistline goals.

Workout: Combine cardio with core work to reap the flat-waistline benefits of both types of sweat sessions. This workout alternates between jumping rope and standing ab moves, so you can tone your waistline while burning serious calories in just 20 minutes.

Day 12

DASH Recipe: Using hydrating honeydew melon for our green juice mocktail gives it a bright, fun hue. A little bit of ginger adds a slight spiciness that also aids with digestion. The recipe serves four, so invite your friends over for a healthy happy hour while you enjoy your rest day.

Workout: Today's workout isn't a workout at all! First up: some well-deserved time away from the gym. While a rest day doesn't have to equal just sitting on the couch, it's important to allow your body time to repair itself — that's how strong, calorie-burning muscles are made. So today, take a time-out with a low-intensity workout like a walk or restorative yoga. Or, just enjoy a relaxing night in. And why not enjoy a fresh, tasty mocktail while you're at it? You've earned it!

Day 13

DASH Recipe: Celebrate Summer and satisfy your sweet tooth with this grain-free crumble featuring blueberries, which studies indicate may fight waistline fat. This dessert also features almonds; high in MUFAs (monounsaturated fats), almonds help burn away the fat that collects around your middle.

Workout: Today's workout is 30 minutes of steady-state cardio followed by some serious ab work. Pick your favorite cardio — running, cycling, swimming, dancing — and keep moving at a steady pace for 30 minutes. Then strengthen your core and tone your abs with a 10-minute video featuring surprising variations of sit-ups and planks.

Day 14

DASH Recipe: With just a few ingredients including red peppers, ground turkey, and tomatoes, in less than 30 minutes, you can create a fresh, clean meal with more than 30 grams of protein! A meal high in protein will satiate your hunger, so you stay satisfied without the urge to reach for a high-calorie late-night treat.

Workout: Skip the crunches and hop on your mat for our effective yoga workout designed to target the abs. Begin with a few Sun Salutations to warm up, and then move through this 14-pose sequence on the right side, and repeat on the left. Keep in mind that solely doing core-strengthening moves like these isn't the key to a flatter stomach, but it is part of the equation. Toned abs will look slimmer once you do lose overall body fat from doing cardio, and having more muscle mass increases your calorie burn.

Day 15

DASH Recipe: If you've been feeling tired and in need of a body boost, prepare our delicious and debloating papaya ginger mint smoothie. With stomach-calming ginger and mint, plus the probiotics in Greek yogurt, it will help relieve digestion and flush out toxins, leaving you feeling refreshed. If you've enjoyed an indulgent weekend, this smoothie is a perfect way to wind down.

Workout: For a quick workout that torches calories, tackle today's 30-minute treadmill interval workout. This boredom-busting workout will burn waistline fat and leave you feeling energized for the week ahead.

Day 16

DASH Recipe: Full of whole-grain fiber, a hearty bowl of oatmeal will fill you up and keep you satisfied all morning, which means no need to snack on high-calorie treats before lunch. Buying plain oats is healthier and less expensive than buying presweetened flavored packets, but making your own doesn't mean you have to go without flavor. Add fruit, nuts, nut butter, flax or chia seeds, pureed frozen fruit, and yogurt to increase the waistline-filling fiber and protein without adding a ton of extra calories.

Workout: Today's workout is all about Tabata. Tabata is high-intensity training that's fun, blasts calories, and moves so quickly that it's hard to get bored. For this type of interval workout, you perform an exercise at maximum intensity for 20 seconds, followed by 10 seconds of rest. You repeat this on-off pattern a total of eight times, making one complete Tabata round four minutes.

Day 17

DASH Recipe: Relieve digestion woes and help shrink your waistline with a tropical pineapple arugula salad. Pineapple contains enzymes that help you debloat and ease digestion, while avocado contains fiber and MUFAs (monounsaturated fatty acids) to fight waistline fat. Plus, this salad is bursting with fresh flavor, so all your taste buds will be satisfied.

Workout: Today's challenge is a waistline-blasting cardio workout — intervals on the treadmill. It's an excellent way to target midsection fat.

Note: Looking for an extra flat-waistline boost today? Add a few detoxing and debloating ingredients to your water. Squeeze some lemon, grate some ginger, and slice some cucumber into your water for added flavor and nutrients. You might even find yourself drinking more — a great strategy for flushing out your system and making you feel less puffy.

Day 18

DASH Recipe: After a tough strength-training session like this bodyweight workout, protein is necessary to help your body recover. And that protein-packed meal needs to come together quickly, before your hunger overwhelms you. This delicious panko-crusted fish dinner takes less than 20 minutes from prep to plate, but the best part is one serving offers more than 36 grams of protein, which can help the body burn more fat!

Workouts: Who needs a gym? With this bodyweight workout, you can tone your entire body anywhere. Our no-equipment workout will get your heart rate up while building metabolism-boosting muscle and whittling your middle. Just print this poster, and get your sweat on anytime you want!

Day 19

DASH Recipe: Relax with a cocktail! For anyone craving a fruity cocktail minus the calories, our variation of a classic tequila bramble makes a great choice. The recipe doesn't contain any store-bought mixers or fruit juice but relies on fresh, seasonal waistline-fat-blasting blackberries and a hint of agave syrup for its sweetness. If you want to enjoy your cocktail alcohol-free, you can omit the tequila and substitute the blackberry liqueur with a splash of berry juice concentrate.

Workout: Today it's time to pull back a bit and allow your body the rest it needs to recharge itself. A rest day is just as important as a workout, and you deserve some time away from the gym.

With that said, it's important to remember that a day of rest doesn't always have to equal inactivity. Opt for some light cardio like a walk around the neighborhood, which will help get the blood flowing to tired muscles. If that doesn't appeal to you, give your body the stretch it needs by flowing through a restorative yoga sequence or just enjoy a relaxing night in.

Day 20

DASH Recipe: You've made it 20 days in, so it's time for a treat! Enjoy a vegan chocolate pudding that tastes decadent but is full of healthy waistline-flattening fats thanks to one surprising ingredient. It's a fast and easy treat you can whip up any time and save for later.

Workout: Today's workout is 30 minutes of steady-state cardio followed by some serious ab work. Pick your favorite cardio — running, cycling, swimming, dancing — and keep moving at a steady pace for 30 minutes. Then tone and tighten your midsection with a 10-minute ab video. No need for weights, so no excuses!

Day 21

DASH Recipe: Eating fish can promote weight loss since lean protein fills you up and sustains your energy, which prevents you from over snacking later. Plus it's a great source of omega-3 fatty acids, which we all could use. If you've never made fish, today's recipe is an incredibly easy one that's low in calories (160!)

and only requires four ingredients. Serve alongside our flat-waistline salad for a light, filling dinner.

Workout: Today's yoga sequence is all about burning your own internal fire through fierce twists and loads of vinyasas. The 11 twisting poses will get all your muscles working — it's the perfect sequence to get things moving.

Fighting Waistline Fat With the DASH Diet

We are all familiar with the old saying "you are what you eat", and this could not be truer than when it comes to achieving and maintaining the ideal weight. Diet is one of the most important weapons in the fight against waistline fat and you can lose weight through dieting alone. Experts estimate that around 80 to 90 percent of the success or failure of fat loss will be attributed to your food intake.

However, diets are not equal to stopping certain foods altogether, and instead we should think about a diet as our attitude towards food. They involve changing the kinds of food we eat, as well as the frequency we eat them and the portion sizes.

Getting a balance of a range of different food groups remains the most important thing. It is not a good idea to make your body deficient in a particular nutrient, and you want your new food intake to be sustainable over an extended period of time. Avoid certain diets that only allow you to eat or drink a very limited amount, and this way you will ensure that you will not only lose weight, but also go on to build a healthy body, fueling it with the right levels of nutrition for a long period of time.

The Five Principles to a Successful Nutrition Plan

1. Adequacy – The amount of food you eat should match your activity level during the day.
2. Balance – Avoid only eating one particular type of food. Aim for a balance across the different food groups.
3. Nutrient Density – Consume more foods that are nutrient-dense, while decreasing your consumption of high-energy, low-nutrient dense foods.

4. Moderation – Moderating your portion sizes will help you to manage your weight better as well as reducing your consumption of foods high in sugar and fat.
5. Variety – Variety is the spice of life, and the same goes for weight loss. Do not allow yourself to eat the same meals, or your weight-loss journey will suddenly seem much harder, as well as being more boring.

What to Eat

The first rule is to simply eat real, whole foods that were grown naturally. Processed foods are often low in nutrition, fibre, and high in sugar, salt, additives and preservatives. These food types are not filling and lead to more cravings and overeating. In addition to this, dry to avoid marketing gimmicks like "low fat" and "made with whole grains", which can often mean very little and may be high in sugar.

Below are some examples of real, whole foods that are especially good for you during the weight loss journey.

Fruits and Vegetables

1. Avocado

When compared to other fruits like apples, avocados have a very low sugar content and this is is great news for the insulin levels. They are rich in monounsaturated fat, which is proven to give an energy boost and strengthen metabolism, making it a great pre-workout snack.

One study even found that people who eat half a fresh avocado decreased their desire to eat by 40 percent for a few hours following it. They would certainly make a great breakfast.

2. Berries

Eating berries is an excellent way to satisfy your sweet tooth without feeling guilty, and in comparison to most other fruits, berries have a relatively low calorie and sugar content. In general, fruit is a good source of dietary fiber when eaten whole, leaving you feeling satiated and slowing down sugar absorption.

If you are not sure how to get more berries into your diet, eat them as a snack, or add them to smoothies or stirred through your morning oatmeal.

3. Apples and Pears

Pears and apples are two of only a handful of fruits that are low in calories and high in fiber. Since they are a rich source of dietary fiber, apples and pears will make you feel full without eating too much. Just be sure to eat the whole fruit, as juice alone lacks the necessary dietary fiber needed to digest and process the sugars properly.

4. Grapefruit

Grapefruit is highly beneficial when it comes to burning waistline fat. It stimulates the production of cholecystokinin, a known hunger suppressant. Additionally, grapefruit lowers the insulin levels of the body, which prevents it from storing fat.

Again, you should always aim to eat the whole fruit as the flesh stores most of the nutrients and contains the fiber you need to digest the fruit's sugars properly.

5. Sweet Potato

Sweet potato's inherent natural sweetness makes it a very appealing ingredient for a range of recipes. It is a rich source of antioxidants and anti-inflammatory nutrients that benefit eyesight, heart and digestive system.

Compared to its close relative the potato, sweet potato has a lower glycemic index, which measures how fast it releases sugar into the bloodstream, so it makes a great substitute. It is another food that is rich in dietary fiber that steadies the pace of digestion and gives enough time for the starches to be converted into simple sugars in the digestive tract.

6. Chili Peppers

Chili peppers have one particular ingredient that suppresses the appetite and burns fat, capsaicin. Capsaicin is responsible for the burning sensation in the mouth when we eat chili, but it also burns fat through a process called thermogenesis, and literally converts food into heat for over 20 minutes after we eat it.

7. Leafy Greens

Leafy greens such as kale, spinach, and romaine lettuce are known for their rich nutrient and fiber content, while being low in carbohydrates and calories. Leafy greens are one of the healthiest foods you can add to your diet because of their low energy density (low calories), meaning you can eat more without much risk of gaining weight. They also help you feel to full for longer.

8. Cruciferous Vegetables

Some of the notable characters in this group are arugula, broccoli, bok choy, collard greens, kale, daikon radish, watercress, radish, turnip, and mustard greens.

This vegetable family is rich in vitamin A, vitamin C, folic acid (a crucial nutrient for pregnant women), carotenoids, and fiber, while also being low in calories and fat.

Per one hundred calories you consume, you will receive around 25 to 40 percent of your daily dietary fiber requirement, this not only helps with weight loss, but also aids in improving digestive health.

Beans and Legumes

Beans and legumes are rare in that they combine high protein and fiber without saturated fat. This is what makes them ideal for moderating or losing weight because protein and fiber go through the digestive system at a slower pace, leaving you feeling fuller for longer, as well as helping to move along any foods that might be stuck in your gastrointestinal tract.

The slower pace also helps regulate the blood sugar balance, and beans also lead to the production of a hormone known to be an appetite suppressant.

Meat and Fish

1. Lean grass-fed beef and organic chicken

Adding lean beef to your diet is one way to help you lose weight because of its protein content. Studies have shown that by simply adding protein to your diet, cravings can be reduced by up to 60 percent.

Chicken breast is another fantastic source of protein which makes it a staple of a lot of weight loss diets. You should aim to grill meat wherever possible, as frying it will add to the calorie content.

2. Wild-caught salmon

Salmon is a rich source of nutrients that indirectly help in regulating weight. This nutrient-dense fish is rich in omega-3 fatty acids which boost brain function and contribute to improving the overall mood. Omega-3 also helps reduce inflammation and aids digestion. Better digestion means better weight regulation, reducing the chances of obesity and metabolic disease.

Studies have also shown that salmon contains proteins and amino acids that affect insulin effectiveness and the inflammation of the digestive tract.

Additional Ingredients

1. Apple Cider Vinegar

For those fond of salads, instead of using fatty or creamy dressings which can make an otherwise healthy dish pretty unhealthy, try using an apple cider vinegar-based vinaigrette instead. Alternatively, you could drink it by diluting it in water.

Apple cider vinegar is rich in acetic acid, which in one study was found to suppress body fat accumulation and, in others, linked to improving insulin sensitivity in people who have type-2 diabetes.

2. Plain Greek Yogurt

This is a healthier alternative to traditional yogurt because it has less sodium, sugar, and carbohydrates, and it also has more protein. Yogurt, in general, is also a rich source of probiotics, a major factor in our digestive health, providing good bacteria.

Be sure to choose plain unflavored and unsweetened Greek yogurt for the optimal results. You can add fruits to sweeten it naturally, or add it to a healthy smoothie recipe.

3. Nuts

Generally speaking, nuts are a rich source of healthy fats (omega-3 fatty acids), protein, and fiber, but not all nuts are the same, as almonds, cashews, and pistachios contain the least amount of calories so are the ones to go for.

Almonds, in particular, are proven to help in weight loss, in one study a 3-ounce almond supplement saw participants lose 7 percent more in terms of body weight, compared to the other group that had a supplement of complex carbohydrates.

Macadamia and pecans contain the most calories so you should certainly try and minimize these in your weight-loss journey.

4. Coconut Oil

Coconut oil is a rich source of fatty acids, which is great for boosting brain function, lowering blood cholesterol, and potentially helping reduce seizures in people who suffer from epilepsy. Additionally, the high fatty acid content in coconut oil is great for appetite suppression. Use it in place of your usual oil when cooking foods as the taste usually is not overpowering. Alternatively, add it to your smoothies.

5. Chia Seeds

These seeds are a rich source of omega-3 fatty acids, calcium, phosphorus, magnesium, and protein. A total of 14 percent of chia seed weight is protein. Chia seeds can easily be mixed into juices, smoothies, cereal, veggies, or yogurt to add a contrasting nutty flavor.

6. Matcha

Matcha literally means, 'powdered tea' and it's a special form of green tea that is usually grown in Japan. Unlike traditional green tea where the leaves are discarded, you consume the entire chlorophyll-rich leaves that have been handpicked, steamed, dried, and ground into a fine green powder.

Matcha contains EGCG (epigallocatechin gallate) a very potent antioxidant. It increases fat oxidation (fat burning) by 33 percent, as well as inhibiting fat cell development.

7. Eat More Fiber

Fiber is not just super healthy for your heart and cholesterol, it is also a stomach toner. A recent study found that foods high in fiber could reduce visceral body fat - the fat cells deep in the Waistline. Researchers say that for every 10-gram increase in soluble fiber eaten every day, visceral fat was reduced by 3.7 percent over five years.

The best places to find soluble fiber is in vegetables, fruit, and beans, so these are all to be encouraged.

What Not to Eat

1. Hold the Salt

Salt is an essential electrolyte, especially if you are working out and perspiring a lot, but you also need to avoid consuming too much of it, as this can lead to water retention, which causes bloating.

Salt is often to be found in packaged or processed foods, so check the nutrition facts label for sodium levels, or do all of your cooking at home and carefully monitor the salt you add to dishes, as well as opting for low-sodium ingredients.

2. Skip the Diet Soda

Any beverages with bubbles will leave you bloated, but some research suggests that diet sodas might lead to increased waistline fat in addition to bloating. Studies found that people who drank diet soda gained almost triple the abdominal fat over nine years, when compared with those who avoided diet soda.

3. Say "No" to Bread, Even Whole Wheat!

Most bread causes a spike in blood sugar followed by a crash, and all without any real nutritional value. Wheat has been found to stimulate hunger. Additionally, most store-bought breads contain hydrogenated oils, artificial sweeteners, high fructose corn syrup, and preservatives. None of which are beneficial to the body.

4. Avoid Refined Carbohydrates

Not all carbohydrates are equal, and while they are generally viewed in a negative light, often the real problem is with refined carbohydrates. Refined carbohydrates are pure sugar, completely stripped of their fiber leaving only simple carbohydrates behind. This makes foods containing them addictive, and emerging research is showing that refined carbohydrates are the real danger behind metabolic damage.

Be wary of carbohydrates in breads, white pastas, and breakfast cereals, and avoid them where possible.

5. Cut the Junk Out

This should go without saying, but the majority of junk foods really are not doing anything helpful for the waistline. In fact, one study showed that for some people with metabolic disease, just one high-calorie milkshake was enough to make it even worse, and in other people, relatively short periods of overeating could trigger the beginnings of metabolic disease.

6. Steer Clear from Processed Foods

So many of the packaged foods we buy from stores have been processed in some way or other. Even supposedly healthy foods, when made on such a large scale, have to be processed in some way or other. This often means adding lots of chemicals that can cause damage to our bodies.

One study from Georgia State University looked at the effects of preservatives on mice. In only 12 weeks, mice that had been fed with emulsifiers (a common preservative used to maintain food texture) ate more food, and gained more weight. Those mice also became glucose intolerant, setting them up for diabetes and metabolic syndrome.

Flavor-enhancing chemicals added to foods to make them more satisfying can also lead to overconsumption and even addiction to these foods.

Drink Recipes to Lose Waistline Fat for Women in Menopause

This recipe combines three ingredients that each work wonders for your body when it comes to weight management. By bringing them together in this delicious drink that can replace your morning coffee, or by drinking it after meals to help aid digestion, you can get the waistline you deserve.

Ingredients:

- One tablespoon of lemon juice
- One teaspoon of cinnamon
- One tablespoon of raw honey

Directions:

Mix these three ingredients with boiling water and drink it first thing in the morning on an empty stomach, or prior to large meals to increase stomach acidity and aid proper digestion.

Lemons help minimize weight gain while also improving insulin resistance in the body. They are high in pectin fiber, which helps keep you feeling full for longer, fighting hunger pangs, and keep cravings at bay.

Raw Honey is a healthy alternative to sugar, and you can use it to sweeten foods and beverages. However, make sure when you're shopping for honey that you don't purchase pasteurized honey, which is void of nutrition. Instead, opt for raw honey, as its beneficial enzymes and antimicrobial properties will still be intact.

Cinnamon can imitate the activity of insulin in the body, regulating blood sugar levels.

Fighting Waistline Fat with the DASH Diet + Exercises

Stomach fat can sometimes seem impossible to get rid of when you are losing weight. It always feels as though it stays where it is, even during the most rigorous exercises. When you first begin exercising, you will start to notice significant changes within the first few months, such as a slimmer face, more defined shoulders and a less flabby back. But stomach fat can be stubborn.

The best tip you will get is to stay positive and keep at it. Do a combination of aerobic workouts and muscle or strength training workouts using weights, as similar to food, variety is vital when exercising. Many people are afraid that working out their muscles might make them "bulky", but in reality, building muscle can give the appearance of being thinner, especially in the stomach area. Toning muscle helps keep the body looking tight and firm.

Further to this, doing only cardio exercise is not a good plan for losing weight. Spending long hours on a treadmill is something of a waste of energy, when strength training can get you results much more quickly. Plus, muscle burns more calories than fat. This may mean that even as you sleep, having a more muscular body will have you burning more calories.

All of this doesn't mean you have to take out an expensive gym membership, though. There are plenty of exercises you can do in the comfort of your own home, without the need for any equipment.

The Home Workout

The following exercises not only burn fat but can help tone muscle too, which is really important for sculpting the ideal body.

The Crunch

The crunch is so simple to do and still proves to be more effective than many abdominal workout devices, or DVDs on offer.

To start off, lay on your back with your knees up and your feet flat on the ground. For an extra challenge, you can have the bottoms of your feet facing each other with your knees out to the side, but if you are just starting out, try keeping your feet flat on the ground.

While laying flat on your back, flex your ab muscles and lift the upper half of your torso as high off of the ground as possible, keeping a straight back. Hold this position for one full second and slowly lower yourself back down to the ground. It should take three seconds in total to complete one repetition, one second going up, holding for one second, and one second going down. Perform at least ten repetitions per set.

Your hand position in this exercise isn't that important, as long as you are feeling tension in your abs. You can have your arms at your sides, or you can cross them over your chest or cup your ears for an extra challenge, just don't "pull" your head up with your hands!

The Plank

The plank is unique because it is an isometric exercise, which means that it is an exercise where you are not moving or performing repetitions. Several studies have found isometric exercises to be especially effective because they raise the temperature of deep muscle tissue.

To make sure you get the most out of the plank, place your elbows under the shoulders, and hold your core tight, like you are bracing for a punch. Be sure your body is in a straight line from the back of your head to your heels, and do not let your hips or shoulders drop. Hold this position for 20-30 seconds, increasing your time as you progress over the weeks.

To add some variation to this exercise, go on one elbow and turn your body to the side, keeping your hips facing the ground. This will work out your obliques (often referred to as love handles), and it will tone the side of your waistline as well as the front. If you want to add this variation, dedicate 10 seconds of your 30-second plank to each side, with the remaining 10 seconds being spent on the original position.

Scissors

This is one of the more complicated moves, but it is a great combination of cardio and muscle building.

Lie on your back with your hands cupping the back of your head. Flexing your abs, bring your left knee up and twist your torso forwards and across, so that the knee touches your right elbow. Then alternate with your right knee touching your left elbow. Your legs should look like they are performing a cycling motion, similar to riding a bike.

Once you have done both sides, count one rep, and aim to complete 10-15 reps.

The Routine

Perform all of these exercises consecutively, at around 30 seconds each, which should take 90 seconds in total. Rest for 30 seconds and repeat at least five or six more times, or until you cannot do the exercises with correct form any longer.

Do not be discouraged if you need to take longer rest periods after the first cycle or two, with a 30-second rest period as a recommendation. You can take up to a minute long break depending on your fitness level. Remember, the aim is to push yourself, but overexerting your body can have a negative effect on your fat loss goals. Over time, work to reduce your resting periods, but there is no need to do this immediately.

This routine can take as little as 10 minutes. This may seem too short to provide any noticeable improvements. However, it is a high-intensity exercise, which many studies have proven to be more effective at burning fat than longer endurance exercises.

Take up Pilates

If crunches are not successful, pilates may be the exercise you are looking for. Sit-ups and crunches only target the outermost abdominal muscles, the rectus abdominis, whereas pilates train the external obliques, the erector spinae, and the transversus abdominis. That last muscle is what keeps the stomach toned.

By working muscles that are deep down in the body, you will start to notice improved core strength as well as tighter-looking muscles. A strong transversus will act similar to a corset, helping to protect against back pain, but also making your stomach appear leaner and flatter. No amount of crunches can deliver the same result.

Most gyms will have classes available, and they are well worth attending. Even if you feel slightly shy at first, being in a fitness class environment can have really positive effects on your workout, as you push yourself further than you might alone and start to feel part of a community of people with a shared goal.

CONCLUSION

You have dedicated yourself to radically alter your lifestyle, together with the final goal of losing weight, and also naturally obtaining a healthy human body. You begin with great courage, however, after a week you start to be aware of all the temptations you face daily.

With all these tips carefully folled and kept in your mind, you will likely feel much more confident to stay on course. Always remember that it requires a great deal of effort, particularly in the very first months. However, after a little while, everything begins to develop into a routine, and this is the point at which you have permanently altered your lifestyle.

You will not think about everything you did before, but appreciate all the benefits. You do not need to cut salt completely out of your diet to have a positive impact on your blood pressure, as pairing decreased sodium with increased potassium has a greater impact that reducing sodium alone. Potassium is found in fruits, vegetables, and legumes. Sodium and potassium work together in many functions of the body, including maintaining the blood pressure. The system works best when your intake of sodium and potassium are balanced, but in this world of processed, fast food, sources of sodium are consumed far more than sources of potassium.

The DASH (Dietary Approaches to Stop Hypertension) Diet is not so much a diet as a balanced way to eat. It focuses on reducing processed foods and refined grains (high amounts of sodium), while simultaneously increasing fruits, vegetables, nuts and whole grains, and plant proteins (high amounts of potassium).

Foods that are great sources of potassium include bananas, raisins, orange, potato, dried beans and peas, salmon, sunflower seeds and yogurt. Opt for fresh foods over canned foods, whenever possible. If you are using canned beans or legumes, look for low-sodium versions and be sure to drain and rinse them thoroughly before using them.

Soups, breads, canned foods and frozen meals are often packed with sodium. The next time you are in the supermarket take a look at the nutrition label and choose the foods with the lowest sodium amounts. The boxes to pay attention to are cereals, crackers, pasta sauces, canned beans and vegetables, and frozen meals. Low sodium on a label means the product has less than 140mg of sodium per serving. Very low sodium means 35mg or less per serving, and salt or sodium-free means less than 5mg sodium per serving, and does not contain sodium chloride.

The research on the relationship between potassium and weight management is so convincing, the FDA has required the amount of potassium per serving to be listed on the newly-revised nutrition label as a percentage of the Recommended Dietary Allowance. Although the new label has not been fully implemented yet, some brands have already made the change. Look at both the sodium and potassium values on processed and packaged food to get a clearer picture of how the food may impact your blood pressure. Take these into consideration when finding where they fit best in relation to the DASH diet.

REFERENCES

1. Kerley CP. Dietary patterns and components to prevent and treat heart failure: a comprehensive review of human studies. Nutr Res Rev. 2018 Aug 16;:1-27. [PubMed]

2. Spence JD. Controlling resistant hypertension. Stroke Vasc Neurol. 2018 Jun;3(2):69-75. [PMC free article] [PubMed]

3. Dominguez LJ, Barbagallo M. Nutritional prevention of cognitive decline and dementia. Acta Biomed. 2018 Jun 07;89(2):276-290. [PMC free article] [PubMed]

4. Kerley CP. A Review of Plant-based Diets to Prevent and Treat Heart Failure. Card Fail Rev. 2018 May;4(1):54-61. [PMC free article] [PubMed]

5. Ozemek C, Laddu DR, Arena R, Lavie CJ. The role of diet for prevention and management of hypertension. Curr. Opin. Cardiol. 2018 Jul;33(4):388-393. [PubMed]

6. Dos Reis Padilha G, Sanches Machado d'Almeida K, Ronchi Spillere S, Corrêa Souza G. Dietary Patterns in Secondary Prevention of

Heart Failure: A Systematic Review. Nutrients. 2018 Jun 26;10(7) [PMC free article] [PubMed]

7. Urrico P. Nonpharmacological Interventions in the Management of Hypertension in the Adult Population With Type 2 Diabetes Mellitus. Can J Diabetes. 2018 Apr;42(2):196-198. [PubMed]

8. Garcia-Rios A, Ordovas JM, Lopez-Miranda J, Perez-Martinez P. New diet trials and cardiovascular risk. Curr. Opin. Cardiol. 2018 Jul;33(4):423-428. [PubMed]

9. Sanches Machado d'Almeida K, Ronchi Spillere S, Zuchinali P, Corrêa Souza G. Mediterranean Diet and Other Dietary Patterns in Primary Prevention of Heart Failure and Changes in Cardiac Function Markers: A Systematic Review. Nutrients. 2018 Jan 10;10(1) [PMC free article] [PubMed]

10. Scisney-Matlock M, Bosworth HB, Giger JN, Strickland OL, Harrison RV, Coverson D, Shah NR, Dennison CR, Dunbar-Jacob JM, Jones L, Ogedegbe G, Batts-Turner ML, Jamerson KA. Strategies for implementing and sustaining therapeutic lifestyle changes as part of hypertension management in African Americans. Postgrad Med. 2009

May;121(3):147-59. [PMC free article] [PubMed]

11. Saneei P, Fallahi E, Barak F, Ghasemifard N, Keshteli AH, Yazdannik AR, Esmaillzadeh A. Adherence to the DASH diet and prevalence of the metabolic syndrome among Iranian women. Eur J Nutr. 2015 Apr;54(3):421-8. [PubMed]

12. Nathenson P. The DASH diet: A cultural adaptation. Nursing. 2017 Apr;47(4):57-59. [PubMed]

13. Wang T, Heianza Y, Sun D, Huang T, Ma W, Rimm EB, Manson JE, Hu FB, Willett WC, Qi L. Improving adherence to healthy dietary patterns, genetic risk, and long term weight gain: gene-diet interaction analysis in two prospective cohort studies. BMJ. 2018 Jan 10;360:j5644. [PMC free article] [PubMed]

14. Mahdavi R, Bagheri Asl A, Abadi MAJ, Namazi N. Perceived Barriers to Following Dietary Recommendations in Hypertensive Patients. J Am Coll Nutr. 2017 Mar-Apr;36(3):193-199.

15. Little T, et al. Role of cholecystokinin in appetite control and body weight regulation. - PubMed - NCBI. Ncbinlmnih.gov. 2016.

Available at: http://www.ncbi.nlm.nih.gov/pubmed/16246215. Accessed August 26, 2016.

16. Blueberries, raw Nutrition Facts & Calories. Nutritiondataself.com. 2016. Available at: http://nutritiondata.self.com/facts/fruits-and-fruit-juices/1851/2. Accessed August 26, 2016.

17. Anderson JW e. Health benefits of dietary fiber. - PubMed - NCBI. Ncbinlmnih.gov. 2016. Available at: http://www.ncbi.nlm.nih.gov/pubmed/19335713. Accessed August 26, 2016.

18. Heini A, et al. Effect of hydrolyzed guar fiber on fasting and postprandial satiety and satiety hormones: A double-blind, placebo-controlled trial during controlled weight loss. Static11sqspcdncom. 1998. Available at: http://static1.1.sqspcdn.com/static/f/746362/21703159/1358792104753/Sunfiber+-+Heini.pdf?token=BQO68UmLOXfUwS8CQjO3%2By%2BsAlY%3D. Accessed August 26, 2016.

19. Fujioka K e. The effects of grapefruit on weight and insulin resistance: relationship to the metabolic syndrome. - PubMed - NCBI. Ncbinlmnih.gov. 2016. Available at:

http://www.ncbi.nlm.nih.gov/pubmed/16579728. Accessed August 26, 2016.

20. Diabetes Superfoods. American Diabetes Association. 2016. Available at: http://www.diabetes.org/food-and-fitness/food/what-can-i-eat/making-healthy-foodchoices/diabetes-superfoods.html?loc=ff-slabnav?referrer=http://www.livestrong.com/article/424496-sweet-potato-and-weight-loss/. Accessed August 26, 2016.

21. Sweet potatoes. Whfoods. 2016. Available at: http://www.whfoods.com/genpage.php?tname=foodspice&dbid=64. Accessed August 29, 2016.

22. 6 Ways Cinnamon Can Aid Weight Loss. IdealBite. 2013. Available at: http://idealbite.com/cinnamon-for-weight-loss/. Accessed August 29, 2016.

23. 2 Pilates Moves for Stronger Abs. SparkPeople. 2016. Available at: http://www.sparkpeople.com/blog/blog.asp?post=2_pilates_moves_for_a_flatter_belly. Accessed August 29, 2016.

58 59

24. How Hidden Food Sensitivities Make You Fat - Dr. Mark Hyman. Dr Mark Hyman. 2012.

Available at: http://drhyman.com/blog/2012/02/22/how-hidden-food-sensitivities-make-you-fat/. Accessed August 29, 2016.

25. Obesity and overweight. World Health Organization. 2016. Available at: http://www.who.int/mediacentre/factsheets/fs311/en/. Accessed August 29, 2016.

26. Epel ES e. Stress and body shape: stress-induced cortisol secretion is consistently greater among women with central fat. - PubMed - NCBI. Ncbinlmnih.gov. 2016. Available at: http://www.ncbi.nlm.nih.gov/pubmed/11020091. Accessed August 31, 2016.

27. Stress Cortisol Connection. Unmedu. 2016. Available at: https://www.unm.edu/~lkravitz/Article%20folder/stresscortisol.html. Accessed August 31, 2016.

28. How Hormones Cause Muffin Top in Women - How to Lose It. Lose Belly Fat Healthier and Faster. 2014. Available at: http://www.losebellyfatberipped.info/hormones-muffin-top-women. Accessed August 31, 2016.

29. Westerterp-Plantenga MS e. Sensory and gastrointestinal satiety effects of capsaicin on food intake. - PubMed - NCBI. Ncbinlmnih.gov. 2016. Available at: http://www.ncbi.nlm.nih.gov/pubmed/15611784. Accessed August 31, 2016.

30. Capsaicin: 7 Powerful Health Benefits of the Stuff that Makes Peppers HOT. Sixwise.com. 2016. Available at: http://www.sixwise.com/newsletters/06/03/29/capsaicin-7-powerful-health-benefits-of-the-stuff-that-makes-peppers-hot-004.htm. Accessed August 31, 2016.

31. Weight loss: Feel full on fewer calories - Mayo Clinic. Mayoclinic.org. 2016. Available at: http://www.mayoclinic.org/healthy-lifestyle/weight-loss/in-depth/weightloss/art-20044318. Accessed August 31, 2016.

32. Eating Healthy with Cruciferous Vegetables. Whfoods.com. 2016. Available at: http://www.whfoods.com/genpage.php?tname=btnews&dbid=126. Accessed August 31, 2016.

33. Weigle D, Breen P, Matthys C et al. A high-protein diet induces sustained reductions in appetite, ad libitum caloric intake, and body weight despite compensatory changes in

diurnal plasma leptin and ghrelin concentrations. The American Journal of Clinical Nutrition. 2005;82(1):41-48. Available at: http://ajcn.nutrition.org/content/82/1/41.abstract. Accessed August 31, 2016.

34. Wall R e. Fatty acids from fish: the anti-inflammatory potential of long-chain omega-3 fatty acids. - PubMed - NCBI. Ncbinlmnih.gov. 2016. Available at: http://www.ncbi.nlm.nih.gov/pubmed/20500789. Accessed August 31, 2016.

35. Lumeng C, Saltiel A. Inflammatory links between obesity and metabolic disease. The Journal of Clinical Investigation. 2011;121(6):2111-2117. Available at: http://www. jci.org/articles/view/57132. Accessed August 31, 2016.

36. Omega-3 fatty acids. University of Maryland Medical Center. 2016. Available at: http://umm.edu/health/medical/altmed/supplement/omega3-fatty-acids. Accessed August 31, 2016.

37. Kondo T e. Vinegar intake reduces body weight, body fat mass, and serum triglyceride levels in obese Japanese subjects. - PubMed - NCBI. Ncbinlmnih.gov. 2016. Available at:

http://www.ncbi.nlm.nih.gov/pubmed/19661687. Accessed August 31, 2016.

38. Johnston C, Kim C, Buller A. Vinegar Improves Insulin Sensitivity to a High-Carbohydrate Meal in Subjects With Insulin Resistance or Type 2 Diabetes. Diabetes Care. 2004;27(1):281-282. Available at: http://care.diabetesjournals.org/content/27/1/281. Accessed August 31, 2016.

39. Greek Style Yogurt 150g=2/3 cup Nutrition Facts & Calories. Nutritiondataself.com. 2016. Available at: http://nutritiondata.self.com/facts/custom/590715/2. Accessed August 31, 2016.

40. Wien M, Sabate J, Ikle D, Cole S, Kandeel F. Almonds vs complex carbohydrates in a weight reduction program. International Journal of Obesity. 2003;27(11):1365. Available at: http://www.nature.com/ijo/journal/v27/n11/full/0802411a.html. Accessed August 31, 2016.

41. Reger MA e. Effects of beta-hydroxybutyrate on cognition in memory-impaired adults. - PubMed - NCBI. Ncbinlmnih.gov. 2016. Available at: http://www.ncbi.nlm.

nih.gov/pubmed/15123336. Accessed August 31, 2016.

42. Assunção ML e. Effects of dietary coconut oil on the biochemical and anthropometric profiles of women presenting abdominal obesity. - PubMed - NCBI. Ncbinlmnih.gov. 2016. Available at: http://www.ncbi.nlm.nih.gov/pubmed/19437058. Accessed August 31, 2016.

43. Sciencedirect.com. 2016. Available at: http://www.sciencedirect.com/science/article/pii/S1474442208700929. Accessed August 31, 2016.

44. McClernon FJ e. The effects of a low-carbohydrate ketogenic diet and a low-fat diet on mood, hunger, and other self-reported symptoms. - PubMed - NCBI. Ncbinlmnih.gov. 2016. Available at: http://www.ncbi.nlm.nih.gov/pubmed/17228046. Accessed August 31, 2016.

45. Mensfitness.com. 2016. Available at: http://www.mensfitness.com/nutrition/whatto-eat/9-foods-that-should-be-in-every-diet. Accessed August 31, 2016.

46. Zemel MB e. Calcium and dairy acceleration of weight and fat loss during

energy restriction in obese adults. - PubMed - NCBI. Ncbinlmnih.gov. 2016. Available at: http://www.ncbi.nlm.nih.gov/pubmed/15090625. Accessed August 31, 2016.

47. Wheat and hunger | Dr. William Davis. Dr William Davis. 2015. Available at: http://www.wheatbellyblog.com/2015/08/wheat-makes-you-hungry/. Accessed August 31, 2016.

48. Hu F. Are refined carbohydrates worse than saturated fat?. The American Journal of Clinical Nutrition. 2010;91(6):1541. Available at: http://www.ncbi.nlm.nih.gov/pmc/articles/PMC2869506/. Accessed August 31, 2016.

49. Authoritynutrition.com. 2016. Available at: https://authoritynutrition.com/9ways-that-processed-foods-are-killing-people/. Accessed August 31, 2016.

50. How Food Preservatives Make You Fat | Bottom Line Inc. Bottom Line Inc. 2015. Available at: http://bottomlineinc.com/how-food-preservatives-make-you-fat/. Accessed August 31, 2016.

51. Even a little is too much: One junk food snack triggers signals of metabolic disease:

Biomarkers that quantify health can help inform prevention strategies for metabolic disease. ScienceDaily. 2016. Available at: https://www.sciencedaily.com/releases/2015/11/151102152735.htm. Accessed August 31, 2016.

52. Honey, Cinnamon And Lemon For Weight Loss. Fitnessrepublic.com. 2016. Available at: https://fitnessrepublic.com/nutrition/healthy-eating/honey-cinnamon-lemon-for-weight-loss.html. Accessed August 31, 2016.

53. Eat, Fast and Live Longer: BBC Horizon 2012. DocumentaryTube. 2016. Available at: http://www.documentarytube.com/videos/eat-fast-and-live-longer-bbc-horizon-2012. Accessed August 31, 2016.

54. Froy O e. Effect of intermittent fasting on circadian rhythms in mice depends on feeding time. - PubMed - NCBI. Ncbinlmnih.gov. 2016. Available at: http://www.ncbi.nlm.nih.gov/pubmed/19041664. Accessed August 31, 2016.

55. Mack SMack S. Is It a Myth That Muscle Burns More Calories Than Fat?. LIVESTRONG.COM. 2016. Available at: http://www.livestrong.com/article/447243-is-

it-amyth-that-muscle-burns-more-calories-than-fat/. Accessed August 31, 2016.

56. AR P. The relationship of body fat content to deep muscle temperature and isometric endurance in man. - PubMed - NCBI. Ncbinlmnih.gov. 2016. Available at: http://www.ncbi.nlm.nih.gov/pubmed/1126131. Accessed August 31, 2016.

57. Patel SR e. Association between reduced sleep and weight gain in women. - PubMed - NCBI. Ncbinlmnih.gov. 2016. Available at: http://www.ncbi.nlm.nih.gov/pubmed/16914506. Accessed August 31, 2016.

58. Why Lack of Sleep Could Be Making You Fatter | Reader's Digest. Reader's Digest. 2011. Available at: http://www.rd.com/health/diet-weight-loss/why-lack-of-sleepcould-be-making-you-fatter/. Accessed August 31, 2016.

59. The Secret To A Flatter Belly Has Nothing To Do With Sit-Ups. Prevention. 2016. Available at: http://www.prevention.com/fitness/how-posture-can-give-your-a-flatter-belly. Accessed August 31, 2016.

60. Blom WA e. Effect of a high-protein breakfast on the postprandial ghrelin response. - PubMed - NCBI. Ncbinlmnih.gov. 2016. Available at: http://www.ncbi.nlm.nih.gov/pubmed/16469977. Accessed August 31, 2016.

61. Stress Tips: Calm Your Mind, Heal Your Body - Dr. Mark Hyman. Dr Mark Hyman. 2010. Available at: http://drhyman.com/blog/2010/05/19/stress-tips-calm-yourmind-heal-your-body/. Accessed August 31, 2016.

62. GYMNEMA: Uses, Side Effects, Interactions and Warnings - WebMD. Webmd.com. 2016. Available at: http://www.webmd.com/vitamins-supplements/ingredientmono-841-gymnema.aspx?activeingredientid=841&activeingredientname=gymnema. Accessed August 31, 2016.

Made in the USA
Middletown, DE
17 August 2019